WORKBOOK

Adventures in Food and Nutrition

Sixth Edition

by
Ryan M. Judge
Family & Consumer Sciences Education Specialist
Educator, Author, and Professional Speaker
Poughkeepsie, New York

Publisher
The Goodheart-Willcox Company, Inc.
Tinley Park, IL
www.g-w.com

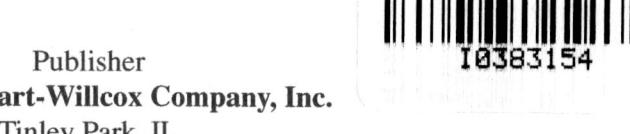

Copyright © 2022
by
The Goodheart-Willcox Company, Inc.

Previous editions copyright 2016, 2012, 2007, 2003, 1997

All rights reserved. No part of this work may be reproduced, stored, or transmitted in any form or by any electronic or mechanical means, including information storage and retrieval systems, without the prior written permission of
The Goodheart-Willcox Company, Inc.

Manufactured in the United States of America.

ISBN: 978-1-63563-853-0

1 2 3 4 5 6 7 8 9 – 22 – 25 24 23 22 21 20

The Goodheart-Willcox Company, Inc. Brand Disclaimer: Brand names, company names, and illustrations for products and services included in this text are provided for educational purposes only and do not represent or imply endorsement or recommendation by the author or the publisher.

The Goodheart-Willcox Company, Inc. Safety Notice: The reader is expressly advised to carefully read, understand, and apply all safety precautions and warnings described in this book or that might also be indicated in undertaking the activities and exercises described herein to minimize risk of personal injury or injury to others. Common sense and good judgment should also be exercised and applied to help avoid all potential hazards. The reader should always refer to the appropriate manufacturer's technical information, directions, and recommendations; then proceed with care to follow specific equipment operating instructions. The reader should understand these notices and cautions are not exhaustive.

The publisher makes no warranty or representation whatsoever, either expressed or implied, including but not limited to equipment, procedures, and applications described or referred to herein, their quality, performance, merchantability, or fitness for a particular purpose. The publisher assumes no responsibility for any changes, errors, or omissions in this book. The publisher specifically disclaims any liability whatsoever, including any direct, indirect, incidental, consequential, special, or exemplary damages resulting, in whole or in part, from the reader's use or reliance upon the information, instructions, procedures, warnings, cautions, applications, or other matter contained in this book. The publisher assumes no responsibility for the activities of the reader.

The Goodheart-Willcox Company, Inc. Internet Disclaimer: The Internet resources and listings in this Goodheart-Willcox Publisher product are provided solely as a convenience to you. These resources and listings were reviewed at the time of publication to provide you with accurate, safe, and appropriate information. Goodheart-Willcox Publisher has no control over the referenced websites and, due to the dynamic nature of the Internet, is not responsible or liable for the content, products, or performance of links to other websites or resources. Goodheart-Willcox Publisher makes no representation, either expressed or implied, regarding the content of these websites, and such references do not constitute an endorsement or recommendation of the information or content presented. It is your responsibility to take all protective measures to guard against inappropriate content, viruses, or other destructive elements.

Cover image: KucherAV/Shutterstock.com

Contents

Chapter 1 Food, Nutrition, and You. 1
- Activity A Laying the Foundation for Wellness . . . 1
- Activity B Tell Your Story 3
- Activity C Oh, Snap! 4
- Activity D New Terms Review 6

Chapter 2 Nutrients: The Building Blocks of Health. 7
- Activity A Two Truths and a Lie 7
- Activity B A Look at Your Plate 9
- Activity C Sorting Nutrients 10
- Activity D Nutrient Friend Profiles 11
- Activity E Advice Emails 12
- Activity F New Terms Review 14

Chapter 3 Your Nutrition Toolbox. 15
- Activity A Find the False News! 15
- Activity B What's on Your Plate? 16
- Activity C Goal Setting 18
- Activity D New (and Other) Terms Review 20

Chapter 4 Weighing Your Choices 21
- Activity A A Tough Balance 21
- Activity B This or That? 22
- Activity C Friendly Advice 23
- Activity D New Terms Review 24

Chapter 5 A Look at the Kitchen 25
- Activity A Oven Organizer 25
- Activity B Range Options 26
- Activity C Find the Truth 27
- Activity D Find Your Center 28
- Activity E New Terms Review 30

Chapter 6 The Cook's Tools. 31
- Activity A Name That Tool 31
- Activity B Name That Appliance 34
- Activity C Should You Buy It? 36
- Activity D New Terms Review 38

Chapter 7 Play It Safe! 39
- Activity A *Un*safe Stanley 39
- Activity B Responding to Accidents 41
- Activity C New Terms Review 42

Chapter 8 Keep It Clean! 43
- Activity A Recognizing the Enemy 43
- Activity B Cleaning Poster Power 44
- Activity C New Terms Review 46

Chapter 9 Recipes—Blueprints for Food . 47
- Activity A A Well-Written Recipe 47
- Activity B Measuring Is off the Charts! 48
- Activity C Am I Making Enough? 49
- Activity D Working with Measurement Equivalents 50
- Activity E Organizing Terms 51
- Activity F New (and Other) Terms Review 52

Chapter 10 What's on the Menu? 53
- Activity A A Blast with Brunch 53
- Activity B Convenience Scavenger Hunt 55
- Activity C New Terms Review 56

Chapter 11 Smart Shopping. 57
- Activity A Where Should They Shop? 57
- Activity B A Smart Shopper Sidekick 59
- Activity C New Terms Review 60

Chapter 12 Ready, Set, Cook! 61
- Activity A Team Time Checklist 61
- Activity B Plan a Party 62
- Activity C New (and Other) Terms Review 64

Chapter 13 Eating on the Go 65
- Activity A Idea Clouds 65
- Activity B Pizza Progress 66
- Activity C Your Lunch-on-the-Go Plan 67
- Activity D Tips and Tips 68

Chapter 14 Fabulous Fruits 69
    Activity A   Fruit Fact or Falsehood? 69
    Activity B   Picture It! 70
    Activity C   Peachy Keen! 71
    Activity D   New Terms Review 72

Chapter 15 Versatile Vegetables 73
    Activity A   Well Versed in Vegetables 73
    Activity B   Vegetable Memes 74
    Activity C   New (and Other) Terms Review 76

Chapter 16 Salad Success 77
    Activity A   Salad Myth Busters 77
    Activity B   Your Ultimate Salad 78
    Activity C   New Terms Review 80

Chapter 17 Great Grains 81
    Activity A   The Nitty-Gritty on Grains 81
    Activity B   Grain Basics 83
    Activity C   Handling Grains 85
    Activity D   New Terms Review 86

Chapter 18 Bountiful Breads 87
    Activity A   Let's Talk Bread! 87
    Activity B   Bread Basics 88
    Activity C   New Terms Review 90

Chapter 19 Luscious Legumes, Nuts, and Seeds 91
    Activity A   Listen Up About Legumes 91
    Activity B   Seeds of Knowledge 93
    Activity C   Advice for a Vegetarian Diet 95
    Activity D   New Terms Review 96

Chapter 20 Dairy Delights 97
    Activity A   Dairy Details 97
    Activity B   Milk Matters 99
    Activity C   Avoiding a Dairy Disaster 101
    Activity D   New Terms Review 102

Chapter 21 Incredible Eggs 103
    Activity A   Beneath the Shell 103
    Activity B   Egg-Handling Intel 105
    Activity C   New Terms Review 106

Chapter 22 Savory Seafood 107
    Activity A   Fishy Business Profiles 107
    Activity B   Name That Cut 109
    Activity C   Seafood Sourcing 110
    Activity D   New (and Other) Terms Review 112

Chapter 23 Marvelous Meat and Poultry 113
    Activity A   Meat and Poultry Basics 113
    Activity B   Handling Meats and Poultry 115
    Activity C   New (and Other) Terms Review 116

Chapter 24 Delicious Desserts 117
    Activity A   Conquering Cake 117
    Activity B   Deciphering Desserts 119
    Activity C   New Terms Review 120

Chapter 25 A Career to Consider 121
    Activity A   Career Reflection 121
    Activity B   Your Vision for a Career 122
    Activity C   New Terms Review 124

Name _____ Date _____ Period _____

CHAPTER 1: Food, Nutrition, and You

Activity A   Lesson 1.1

Laying the Foundation for Wellness

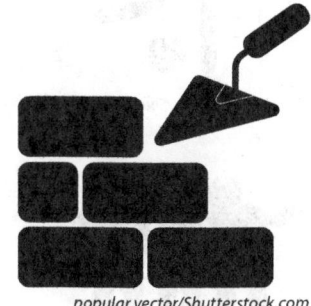
popular.vector/Shutterstock.com

In addition to being delicious, food serves a very important role in people's lives. Answer questions 1–6 using content from the reading.

1. Define *diet*.
   _____
   _____
   _____

2. Define *nutrition*.
   _____
   _____
   _____

3. Define *nutrient*.
   _____
   _____
   _____

4. Define *wellness*.
   _____
   _____
   _____

5. What are three reasons that a nutritious diet is important to a person's wellness?
   _____
   _____
   _____

6. What role does physical activity play in a person's wellness?
   _____
   _____
   _____

(Continued)

Name _____ Date _____ Period _____

Reflect on your personal wellness and rate yourself on a scale of 1–5 (1 is low and 5 is high) for each wellness factor that follows. Provide an explanation for each rating.

7. Physical wellness rating: _____ Explanation:
_____
_____
_____
_____
_____

Best Vector Elements/Shutterstock.com

8. Social wellness rating: _____ Explanation:
_____
_____
_____
_____
_____

Leremy/Shutterstock.com

9. Emotional wellness rating: _____ Explanation:
_____
_____
_____
_____
_____

notbad/Shutterstock.com

10. Intellectual wellness rating: _____ Explanation:
_____
_____
_____
_____
_____

MapensStudio/Shutterstock.com

11. Philosophical wellness rating: _____ Explanation:
_____
_____
_____
_____
_____

johavel/Shutterstock.com

12. Career wellness rating: _____ Explanation:
_____
_____
_____
_____
_____

edel/Shutterstock.com

Name _____ Date _____ Period _____

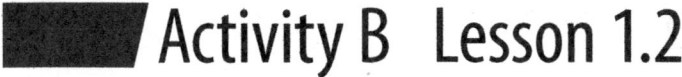 Activity B Lesson 1.2

Tell Your Story

In Lesson 1.2, you read about the factors that affect food choices. In this activity, you will tell your story about the influences on food choices in your life.

For each section in the diagram, compose a one- to two-sentence example of how that particular factor has or does impact your food choices. Be specific. For example, if your family always eats a certain food item on a holiday, place that example under "Family Customs."

Factors That Affect Your Food Choices

Personal Likes

_____
_____
_____
_____
_____

Knowledge

_____
_____
_____
_____
_____

Environment

_____
_____
_____
_____
_____

Culture

_____
_____
_____
_____
_____

Family Customs

_____
_____
_____
_____
_____

Lifestyle

_____
_____
_____
_____
_____

Giant Stock/Shutterstock.com

Name _____ Date _____ Period _____

Activity C Lesson 1.2

Oh, Snap!

Food marketing is everywhere. It is in your school, in your neighborhood, along the streets, in the supermarket, and on TV. In this activity, you will look for examples of food marketing in your life and reflect on its impact.

Step 1. Identify one real-life example of food marketing you observe over the course of your day. Describe the example here.

_____
_____
_____

Step 2. Using the space provided, answer the following questions about the example of food marketing you found.

1. What was being marketed?
   _____
   _____
   _____

2. How was it being marketed?
   _____
   _____
   _____
   _____
   _____

3. Where was it being marketed?
   _____
   _____
   _____
   _____

4. Why do you think the company chose to market its product or company in that way?
   _____
   _____
   _____
   _____

Alexdndz/Shutterstock.com

(Continued)

Name _____ Date _____ Period _____

5. Who do you think the company was targeting through that type of marketing? Explain your answer.
   _____
   _____
   _____
   _____
   _____
   _____
   _____

6. Do you think this marketing is impactful? Explain your answer.
   _____
   _____
   _____
   _____
   _____
   _____
   _____

7. Was it easy or hard for you to find an example of food marketing in your everyday life? Why?
   _____
   _____
   _____
   _____
   _____
   _____
   _____
   _____

8. What did you learn while doing this activity that surprised you?
   _____
   _____
   _____
   _____
   _____
   _____
   _____

Alexdndz/Shutterstock.com

Name _____ Date _____ Period _____

Activity D Chapter 1

New Terms Review

Read each definition and indicate which term is being described.

Definitions

1. _____ The physical need for food.
2. _____ Being at the highest level of health.
3. _____ The knowledge, beliefs, religion, and traditions shared by a group of people.
4. _____ The study of nutrients and how the body uses them.
5. _____ A practice a group of people do often.
6. _____ The materials found in foods that are needed to build and repair body tissues and provide energy.
7. _____ The study of how foods change chemically through natural processes or when they are prepared or stored.
8. _____ A community that has limited access to a variety of healthy foods.
9. _____ A community that has many restaurants offering mostly high-calorie foods at low prices and few fruits, vegetables, and reduced-fat dairy products.
10. _____ All the foods and beverages a person consumes; also referred to as an *eating pattern*.
11. _____ Your surroundings and all the experiences you have.
12. _____ The type of life you lead.
13. _____ A diet that includes energy and all the nutrients in the amounts needed.
14. _____ Any type of action that a company takes to get you to buy their food.
15. _____ The desire to eat certain foods and reject others.

Terms

A. appetite
B. culture
C. custom
D. diet
E. environment
F. food desert
G. food marketing
H. food science
I. food swamp
J. hunger
K. lifestyle
L. nutrients
M. nutrition
N. nutritious diet
O. wellness

Name _____ Date _____ Period _____

CHAPTER 2 — Nutrients: The Building Blocks of Health

Activity A   Lesson 2.1

Two Truths and a Lie

There are many misconceptions about health, wellness, and nutrition. Having a solid foundation of knowledge about nutrients will help you to build healthy habits over your lifetime. Each of the following sets of three statements contains two statements that are true and one statement that is a lie, or is false. In this activity, you will select the statement that is false.

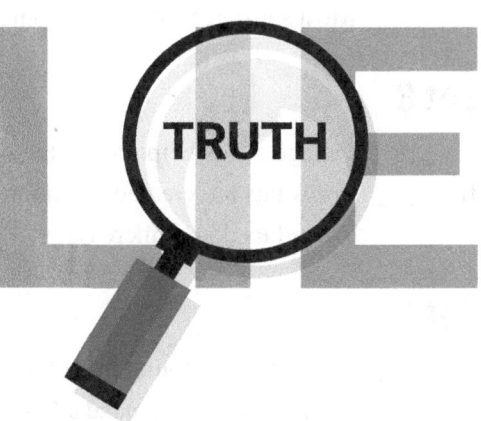

Bakhtiar Zein/Shutterstock.com

Set 1

A. _____ Calories are the form of energy our body needs to function.
B. _____ We get calories from carbohydrate, fat, and protein.
C. _____ Calories are bad for us, and therefore we do not need them.

Set 2

A. _____ Everyone needs the same amount of calories.
B. _____ Carbohydrates have less calories than fat.
C. _____ A gram is a measurement of weight.

Set 3

A. _____ Water is a nutrient.
B. _____ Nutrients do not provide energy.
C. _____ Protein is one of the six classes of nutrients.

Set 4

A. _____ Water is a macronutrient.
B. _____ We need macronutrients in large amounts.
C. _____ We need micronutrients in smaller amounts.

Set 5

A. _____ Carbohydrates can be found in fruits, vegetables, breads, cereals, and milk.
B. _____ Saccharides and sugars are the same thing.
C. _____ All carbohydrates are the same.

(Continued)

Copyright Goodheart-Willcox Co., Inc.
May not be reproduced or posted to a publicly accessible website.

Name _____ Date _____ Period _____

Set 6

A. _____ Starch is a type of carbohydrate.
B. _____ Starch is a complex carbohydrate.
C. _____ Starch should provide the smallest portion of calories in your diet.

Set 7

A. _____ Unsaturated fat causes blood fat and cholesterol levels to rise.
B. _____ Both saturated fats and unsaturated fats provide the same calories per gram.
C. _____ Most saturated fats come from animal sources and most unsaturated fats come from plant sources.

Set 8

A. _____ Omega-3 fats help protect the body from health problems like heart disease and arthritis.
B. _____ *Trans* fats are created by adding hydrogen to an unsaturated fat.
C. _____ *Trans* fats do not increase your risk for heart disease.

Set 9

A. _____ Cholesterol is found in all foods of animal origin.
B. _____ Your body cannot make all the cholesterol it requires, therefore you need to include it in your diet.
C. _____ Proteins are used to build new cells and to repair or replace worn out or damaged cells.

Set 10

A. _____ Food from animals contains all the amino acids you need.
B. _____ You can make incomplete proteins into complete proteins by combining them with each other.
C. _____ Extra protein is stored as muscle.

In the space provided, compose your own two truths and a lie based on content from Lesson 2.1. Indicate the statement that is a lie, or is false.

Set 11

A. _____ _____
B. _____ _____
C. _____ _____

Set 12

A. _____ _____
B. _____ _____
C. _____ _____

Set 13

A. _____ _____
B. _____ _____
C. _____ _____

Name _____ Date _____ Period _____

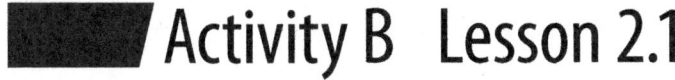 **Activity B   Lesson 2.1**

A Look at Your Plate

One meal does not always give an accurate picture of a person's complete diet, but it is a good start. In the United States, dinner is often the largest meal of the day. In this activity, you will take a closer look at the foods you eat for a typical dinner.

Recall all the foods you consumed during your most recent dinner (including beverages). Organize the foods by category in the chart below based on the nutrients found in each item. (Some foods may be placed in multiple categories if appropriate.) Then summarize your findings below.

Category	Food Item
Carbohydrate	
Saturated Fat	
Unsaturated Fat	
Complete Protein	
Vitamins and Minerals	

Did the results of this activity surprise you? Are there categories you would like to improve? Summarize your findings below.

_____

_____

_____

_____

Name _____ Date _____ Period _____

Activity C Lesson 2.2

Sorting Nutrients

Select the term(s) that belongs in each category.

Category 1: Water-Soluble Vitamins			
Thiamin	Vitamin D	Water	Vitamin A
Vitamin E	Vitamin K	B Vitamins	Calories
Vitamin C	Folate	Niacin	Riboflavin

Category 2: Fat-Soluble Vitamins			
Thiamin	Vitamin D	Water	Vitamin A
Vitamin E	Vitamin K	B Vitamins	Calories
Vitamin C	Folate	Niacin	Riboflavin

Category 3: Micronutrients Lacking in US Diets			
Potassium	Vitamin D	Iron	Vitamin A
Vitamin E	Calcium	B Vitamins	Calories
Vitamin C	Folate	Niacin	Zinc

Category 4: Micronutrients in Excess in US Diets			
Potassium	Vitamin D	Iron	Vitamin A
Sodium	Calcium	B Vitamins	Calories
Vitamin C	Folate	Niacin	Zinc

Name _____ Date _____ Period _____

Activity D Lesson 2.2

Nutrient Friend Profiles

Your "friends"—named *Phytonutrients*, *Water*, and *Antioxidants*—want to meet new people. In this activity, you will create appealing friend profiles for your "friends" to encourage others to get to know them. Create a profile for each "friend" by writing a three- to four-sentence description in the space provided.

davooda/Shutterstock.com

Phytonutrients

_____
_____
_____
_____
_____
_____
_____

Water

_____
_____
_____
_____
_____
_____
_____

Antioxidants

_____
_____
_____
_____
_____
_____
_____
_____

Name _____ Date _____ Period _____

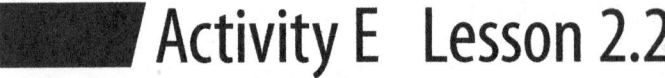 Activity E Lesson 2.2

Advice Emails

Read each of the following emails from people seeking advice. Using your knowledge from the chapter, provide advice for each person based on his or her situation. Place your response in the space provided.

From: Julia Ann <julia@helpme.vit>

To: Family & Consumer Sciences Student Expert <FCS@student.me>

Subject: Vitamins? Are You for Real?

Hey There Student Expert!

My name is Julia Ann and I am 16 years old. I play softball and basketball regularly. My mom bugs me every morning to take a multivitamin supplement. I do not think I need to take one because I feel fine, I'm young, and I am not overweight. However, I cannot get her off my back about it. Based on your knowledge of food and nutrition, do you think I should take one? If so, why? If not, tell me what I can tell my mom so she leaves me alone about it.

Thanks,
Julia

From: Family & Consumer Sciences Student Expert <FCS@student.me>

To: Julia Ann <julia@helpme.vit>

Subject: RE: Vitamins? Are You for Real?

Dear Julia Ann,

_____
_____
_____
_____
_____
_____
_____
_____
_____
_____
_____
_____
_____
_____
_____
_____
_____

Best,
Student Expert

(Continued)

Name _____ Date _____ Period _____

From: Jose Brown <jbrown@helpme.vit>

To: Family & Consumer Sciences Student Expert <FCS@student.me>

Subject: Is Salt Really That Bad?

Hi Student Expert,

I'm Jose Brown and I am 13 years old. My parents work a lot and do not have time to cook big meals. They do buy plenty of fruits, vegetables, bread, cheese, and other healthy food items for me to eat. However, it is annoying to have to put together my meals. Therefore, I like to buy microwavable frozen meals, canned items, etc. that I can just stick in the microwave and heat up. My parents do not want to buy them for me all the time because they say those foods are too high in sodium. I told them I do not care, but they still will not buy them for me. Is a lot of sodium really that bad for me? What should I do?

Thanks,
Jose

From: Family & Consumer Sciences Student Expert <FCS@student.me>

To: Jose Brown <jbrown@helpme.vit>

Subject: RE: Is Salt Really That Bad?

Dear Jose,

_____
_____
_____
_____
_____
_____
_____
_____
_____
_____
_____
_____
_____
_____
_____
_____
_____

Best,
Student Expert

Name _____ Date _____ Period _____

Activity F Chapter 2

New Terms Review

Read each definition and indicate which term is being described.

Definitions

1. _____ A nutrient that provides energy; found in every food of plant origin.
2. _____ A nutrient that provides energy; found in foods of both plant and animal origin.
3. _____ A type of nutrient needed for growth and repair of the body; made of amino acids.
4. _____ A nutrition expert.
5. _____ Types of nutrients that are organic substances needed in small amounts by the body to function, grow, and repair itself.
6. _____ Special proteins that control chemical reactions.
7. _____ Compounds that work together with vitamins, minerals, and fiber to promote good health.
8. _____ A measure of weight.
9. _____ A nutrient that does not provide energy and is needed in only very small amounts each day; vitamins and minerals are examples.
10. _____ Special nutrients and other substances that protect the body's cells from damage that can be caused by oxygen.
11. _____ Types of nutrients that are inorganic substances needed in small amounts by the body to function, grow, and repair itself.
12. _____ A set of guidelines for the amounts of nutrients needed each day.
13. _____ A measure of the energy value of food.
14. _____ A nutrient that provides energy and is needed in large amounts each day; carbohydrates, fats, and proteins are examples.

Terms

A. antioxidants
B. calorie
C. carbohydrate
D. Dietary Reference Intakes (DRIs)
E. dietitian
F. enzymes
G. fat
H. gram
I. macronutrient
J. micronutrient
K. minerals
L. phytonutrients
M. protein
N. vitamins

Name _____ Date _____ Period _____

CHAPTER 3: Your Nutrition Toolbox

Activity A   Lesson 3.1

Find the False News!

Select the term(s) or phrase(s) that belong in each category.

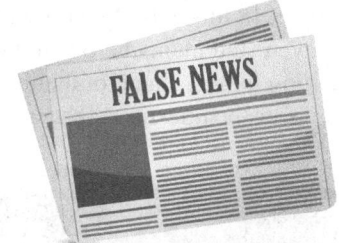
alexmillos/Shutterstock.com

Category 1: *Dietary Guidelines*

Support healthy eating patterns for all.	Be physically active every day.	Eliminate protein from your diet.
Skip meals whenever possible.	Follow a healthy eating pattern across the lifespan.	Only consume foods that are purchased from a health-food store.
Limit calories from added sugars and saturated fats and reduce sodium intake.	Only eat foods that are green.	Shift to healthier food and beverage choices.
Eat large portions of healthy foods every day.	Follow a low-carb diet plan as shown on TV.	Focus on variety, nutrient density, and amount.

Category 2: Nutrient-Dense Foods

Apples	Cake	Carrots
Whole-grain bread	Low-fat yogurt	Soda
Potato chips	Chicken	Beans
Cookies	Sugar-sweetened breakfast cereal	Oatmeal

Category 3: Empty-Calorie Foods

Apples	Cake	Carrots
Whole-grain bread	Low-fat yogurt	Soda
Potato chips	Chicken	Beans
Cookies	Sugar-sweetened breakfast cereal	Oatmeal

Copyright Goodheart-Willcox Co., Inc.
May not be reproduced or posted to a publicly accessible website.

Name _____ Date _____ Period _____

Activity B   Lesson 3.2

What's on Your Plate?

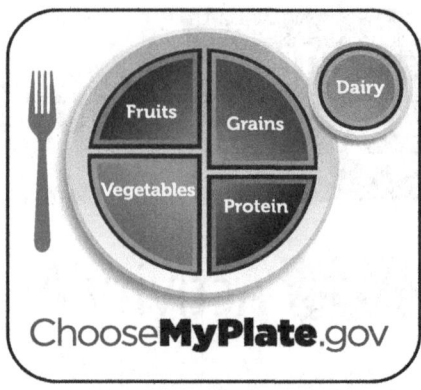

The food decisions you make today can affect your health for years to come. In this activity, you will reflect on your eating habits. For each of the eleven statements below, indicate the frequency that best reflects your current eating habits. Then total and enter your points at the bottom of the chart and answer the questions that follow.

Statement	Frequency			
	Daily (3 points)	Semi-weekly (2 points)	Weekly (1 point)	Never (0 points)
1. I eat breakfast, lunch, and dinner.				
2. I eat whole-grains foods.				
3. I eat fruit.				
4. I eat low-fat or fat-free dairy or calcium-fortified dairy alternative products.				
5. I eat meat, seafood, or a meat substitute such as tofu.				
6. I eat dark green vegetables.				
7. I eat red and orange vegetables.				
8. I eat starchy vegetables.				
9. I eat beans and peas.				
10. I eat other vegetables.				
11. I drink water.				

Your Total Points: _____

In general, the higher your total points, the healthier your eating habits may be. If your total points are greater than 28, you are probably getting many of the nutrients your body needs. However, other factors are also important such as the amounts of these foods being eaten and how much salt, added sugar, and saturated fat are used in their preparation.

(Continued)

Name _____ Date _____ Period _____

Nutritious eating habits are essential to long-term health. Analyze your results by answering the following questions.

12. Are the protein foods you eat largely from animal sources or plant sources? How often do you eat fish or seafood?

_____

_____

_____

13. Many Americans fail to include enough vegetables in their diet. How do the amounts and types of vegetables you eat compare with the amounts identified in Figure 3.13?

_____

_____

_____

_____

_____

14. Oils are not a food group, but they are important for good health. What are the main sources of fat in your diet? Indicate whether the fat is saturated or unsaturated.

_____

_____

_____

_____

_____

15. Overall, how do your results compare with recommendations from the *Dietary Guidelines* and the MyPlate food guidance system? Explain your answer.

_____

_____

_____

_____

_____

16. List two aspects of your eating habits that are healthy for the long-term.

_____

_____

_____

_____

17. List two aspects of your eating habits that you think need improvement.

_____

_____

_____

_____

Name _____ Date _____ Period _____

Activity C   Lesson 3.2

Goal Setting

Setting goals is an effective way to achieve success in all areas of life, including improving one's eating habits. An effective way to set goals is to create SMART goals. SMART goals are *S*pecific, *M*easurable, *A*chievable, *R*elevant, and *T*imely. The following is an example of a SMART goal: Drink three 8-ounce glasses of low-fat or fat-free milk daily for one month.

For this activity, set three SMART goals for your diet. Your answers in Activity B might be a good source of ideas for your goals. For each goal, include at least one positive effect that achieving your goal will have for your health and one possible negative effect that could result if you never changed this eating habit. Then identify one action step to help you achieve each goal.

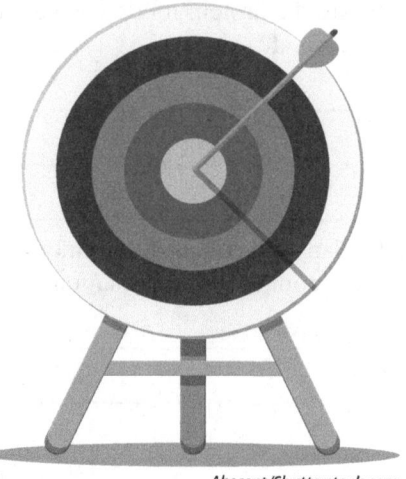
Abscent/Shutterstock.com

SMART Goal #1	Positive Effect(s)	Negative Effect

Identify one action step you will take to help you achieve your first goal.

_____

_____

(Continued)

18   Adventures in Food and Nutrition Workbook

Copyright Goodheart-Willcox Co., Inc.
May not be reproduced or posted to a publicly accessible website.

Name _____ Date _____ Period _____

SMART Goal #2	Positive Effect(s)	Negative Effect

Identify one action step you will take to help you achieve your second goal.

_____

_____

SMART Goal #3	Positive Effect(s)	Negative Effect

Identify one action step you will take to help you achieve your third goal.

_____

_____

Name _____ Date _____ Period _____

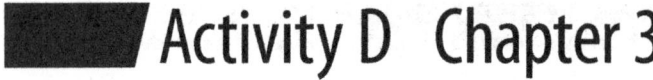 Activity D Chapter 3

New (and Other) Terms Review

Read each definition and indicate which term is being described.

Definitions

1. _____ An image that reminds you how to build a healthy plate and nutritious diet.
2. _____ Foods in this group are good sources of starch, fiber, thiamin, riboflavin, niacin, folic acid, and iron.
3. _____ A type of fat that is essential for health.
4. _____ Foods in this group are low in calories and fat and are rich sources of vitamins such as A and C and folic acid. They also provide phytonutrients, fiber, and minerals such as iron, potassium, and magnesium.
5. _____ Foods in this group are rich sources of protein and calcium, but many contain large amounts of saturated fat and cholesterol. Many also provide vitamin D.
6. _____ Foods that provide small amounts of vitamins, minerals, and other substances needed for good health compared to their calories.
7. _____ A set of recommendations that provides science-based advice to help you choose a nutritious diet and healthful lifestyle.
8. _____ Foods that provide a large amount of vitamins, minerals, and other substances that are needed for good health compared to their calories.
9. _____ Foods in this group supply protein, B vitamins, iron, and zinc. Most of these foods contain large amounts of fat and some contain cholesterol.
10. _____ Sweetens food without adding calories.
11. _____ Foods in this group provide vitamins A and C and potassium. They are low in fat and sodium and provide fiber.

Terms

A. dairy group
B. *Dietary Guidelines for Americans*
C. empty-calorie foods
D. fruit group
E. grains group
F. MyPlate
G. nutrient-dense foods
H. omega-3
I. protein foods group
J. sugar substitute
K. vegetable group

Name _____ Date _____ Period _____

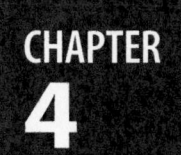
CHAPTER 4
Weighing Your Choices

Activity A   Lesson 4.1

A Tough Balance

Select the correct outcome for the following images.

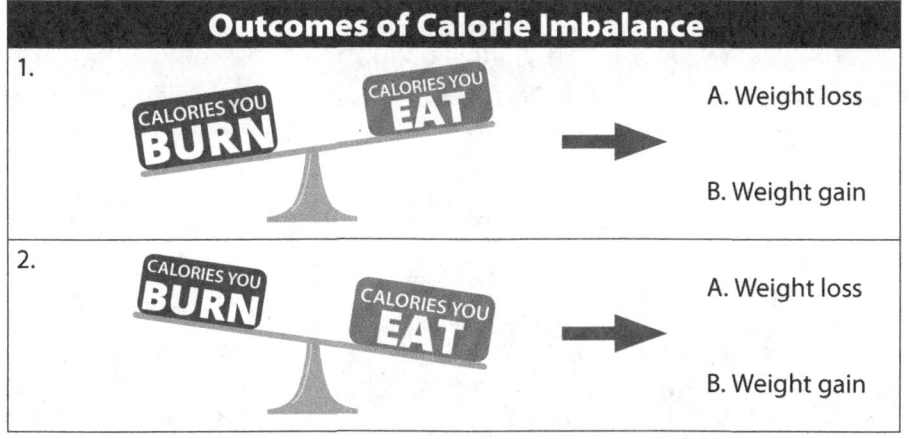

Rudie Strummer/Shutterstock.com

In the chart below, list the health risks associated with each condition.

Overweight	Underweight

Copyright Goodheart-Willcox Co., Inc.
May not be reproduced or posted to a publicly accessible website.

Name _____ Date _____ Period _____

 **Activity B Lesson 4.1**

This or That?

Use the information that follows to answer 1–5 below. You may wish to do your math on a scrap piece of paper.

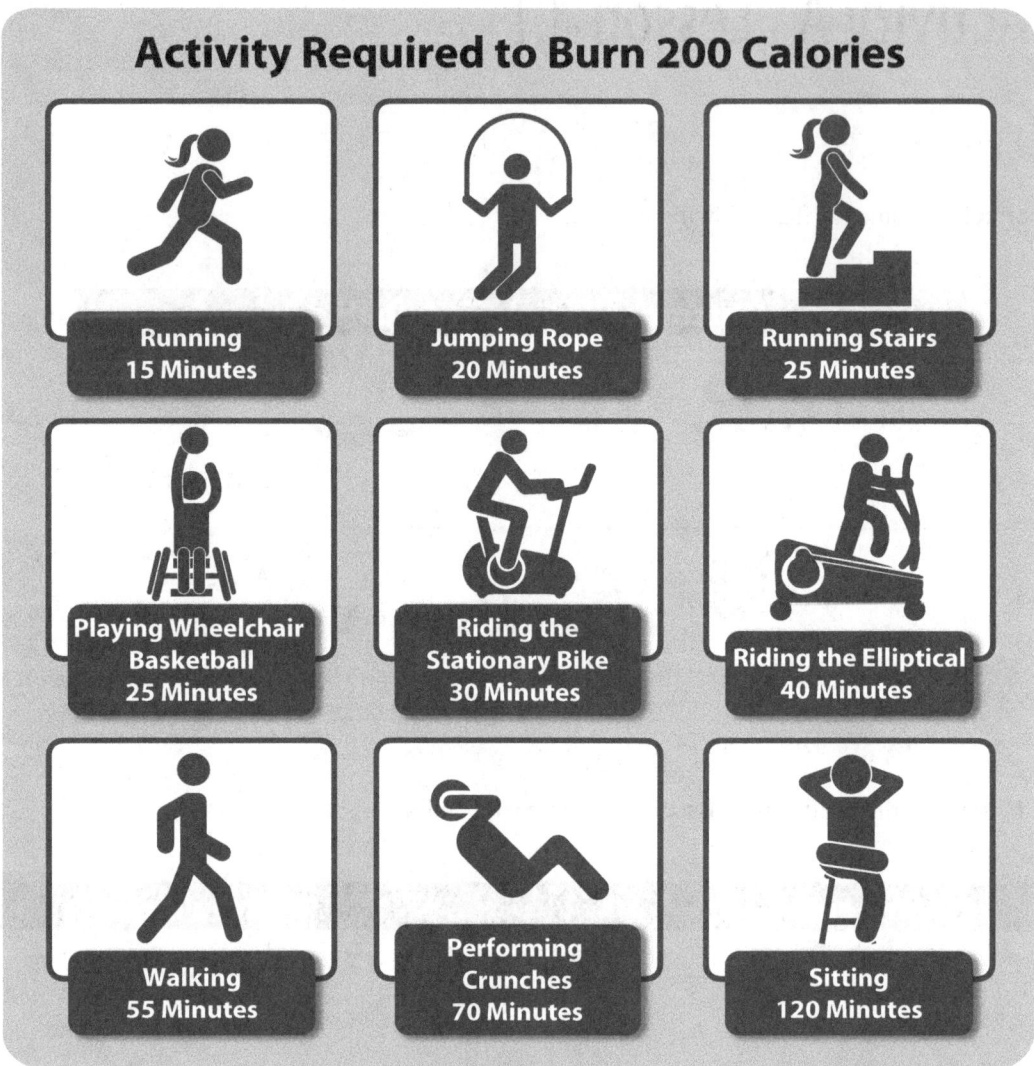

Select the activity from each of the followings pairs that burns more calories:		
1. 30 minutes of walking	or	60 minutes on the elliptical
2. 30 minutes on the stationary bike	or	30 minutes of walking
3. 30 minutes of crunches	or	30 minutes of jumping rope
4. 60 minutes of sitting	or	25 minutes of wheelchair basketball
5. 20 minutes of stair running	or	20 minutes of jumping rope

Name _____ Date _____ Period _____

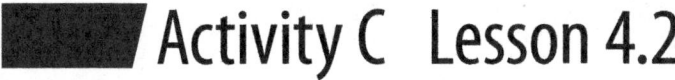 Activity C Lesson 4.2

Friendly Advice

Read the following scenario. Using knowledge from the chapter, provide advice to your friend. The advice should include information about the possible effects of eating disorders and advice on how to prevent an eating disorder.

Scenario

Your friend Dakota recently moved to another state. You and Dakota have been friends since kindergarten, and you know everything about each other. You trust each other more than anyone else in the world. Based on comments during phone calls, images and comments posted on social media, and your knowledge of Dakota's personality, you are worried that Dakota is showing signs of an eating disorder due to the pressures of trying to fit in.

Dear Dakota,

_____
_____
_____
_____
_____
_____
_____
_____
_____
_____
_____
_____
_____
_____
_____
_____
_____
_____
_____
_____
_____
_____
_____
_____
_____

Name _____ Date _____ Period _____

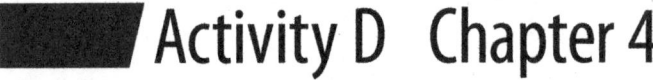 Activity D   Chapter 4

New Terms Review

Read each definition and indicate which term is being described.

Definitions

1. _____ The weight that is right for your age and height.
2. _____ A condition in which people have a weight that is much lower than a healthy weight.
3. _____ A medical condition in which people have an excessive amount of body fat and weigh much more than is healthy.
4. _____ Keeping your body at a healthy weight.
5. _____ A quick weight-loss diet that does not usually work and can harm your health.
6. _____ Abnormal eating practices that are unhealthy.
7. _____ A medical condition such as binge-eating disorder, bulimia nervosa, and anorexia nervosa.
8. _____ A medical condition in which people binge eat.
9. _____ To rapidly consume large quantities of food in a short time for reasons other than hunger.
10. _____ A medical condition in which people binge eat, then compensate using inappropriate behaviors, such as vomiting, fasting, excessively exercising, or misusing medications.
11. _____ A medical condition in which people fear gaining weight and restrict calories so much that they become underweight.

Terms

A. anorexia nervosa
B. binge eat
C. binge-eating disorder
D. bulimia nervosa
E. disordered eating
F. eating disorder
G. fad diet
H. healthy weight
I. obesity
J. underweight
K. weight control

Name _____ Date _____ Period _____

CHAPTER 5 — A Look at the Kitchen

 Activity A   Lesson 5.1

Oven Organizer

Use the graphic organizer below to compare and contrast oven types. Place characteristics that the three ovens share in the center triangle and place the characteristics that are unique to each oven in their respective triangles.

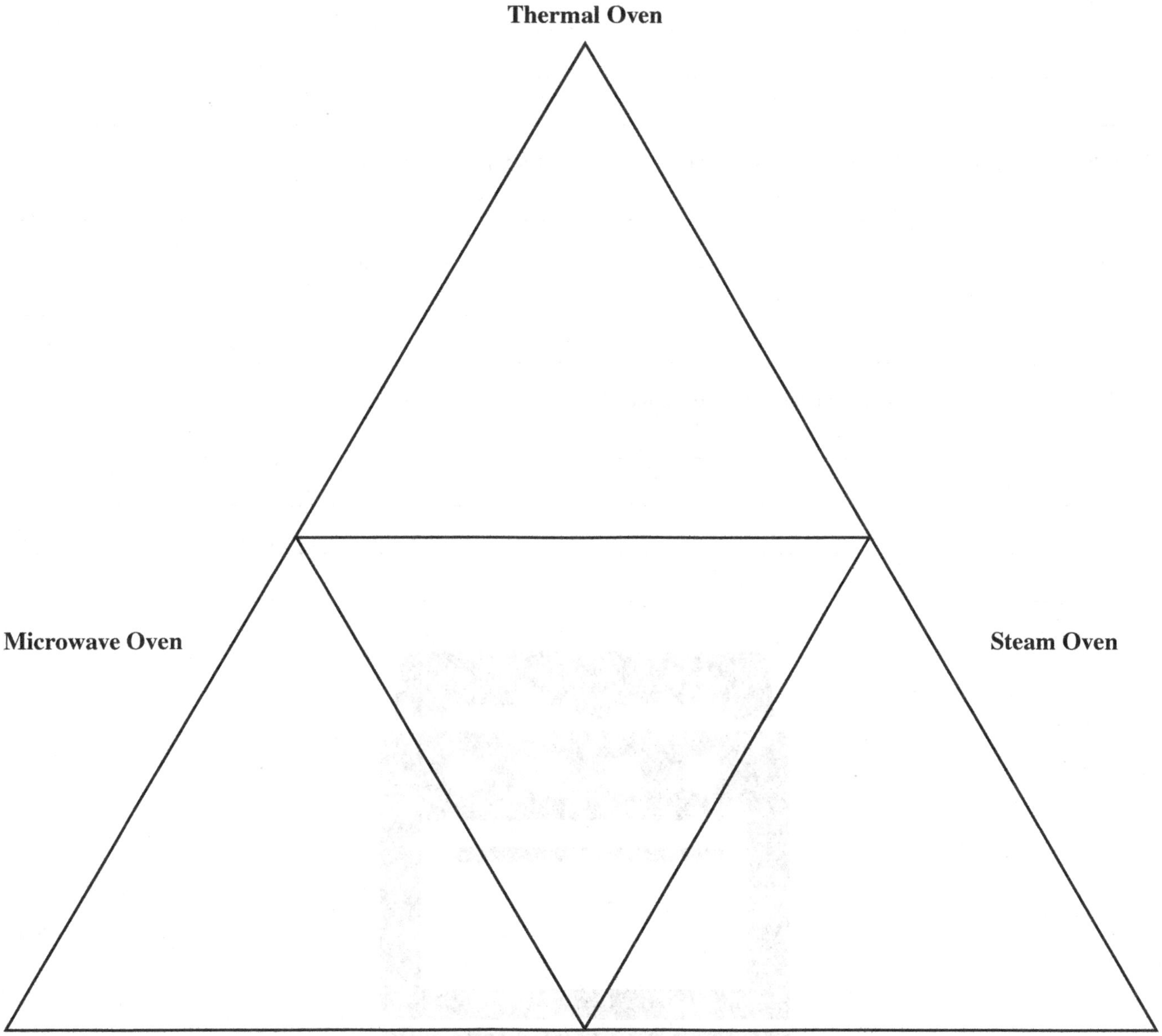

Thermal Oven

Microwave Oven   **Steam Oven**

Name _____ Date _____ Period _____

Activity B   Lesson 5.1

Range Options

1. Imagine you are going to remodel your home kitchen. Which range style would you select? Explain your answer.
   _____
   _____
   _____
   _____

2. What type of oven would you choose? Explain your answer.
   _____
   _____
   _____
   _____

3. What type of fuel would you choose to power your range? Explain your answer.
   _____
   _____
   _____
   _____

4. Describe how to best clean and care for your range choice.
   _____
   _____
   _____
   _____

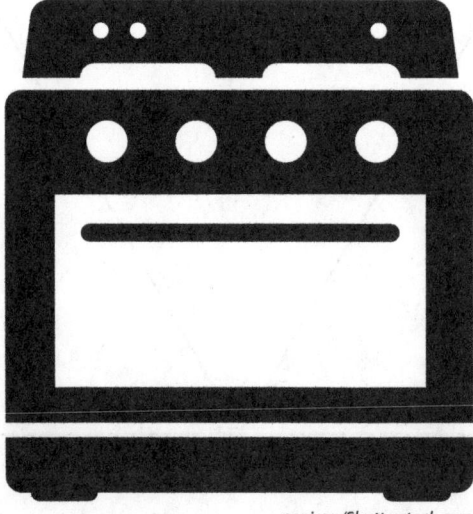

popicon/Shutterstock.com

Name _____ Date _____ Period _____

Activity C   Lesson 5.2

Find the Truth

Indicate whether each statement is true or false.

1. _____ The cold temperatures of a refrigerator or freezer slow the growth of harmful bacteria.
2. _____ Refrigerators and freezers do *not* keep foods fresh longer than if they were stored at room temperature.
3. _____ Before the 1920s, people had to rely on ice or snow to cool foods.
4. _____ Almost all refrigerator styles include a freezer.
5. _____ The temperature of the refrigerator compartment is colder than in the freezer.
6. _____ Chest freezers stay colder than upright freezers because less cold air escapes when they are opened.
7. _____ Chest freezers are best for storing large, bulky packages.
8. _____ Upright freezers are best for storing smaller packages.
9. _____ Frost should be allowed to build up in freezers.
10. _____ Placing an open box of baking soda in the refrigerator absorbs odors and keeps the refrigerator smelling fresh.
11. _____ Dust buildup on the coils at the back of the refrigerator helps the appliance to work more efficiently.
12. _____ How a frozen or refrigerated food item is wrapped does not affect its storage shelf life.
13. _____ The temperatures of the refrigerator and freezer do not affect the food storage shelf life.
14. _____ Dishwashers are self-cleaning.
15. _____ Any type of detergent can be used in a dishwasher.

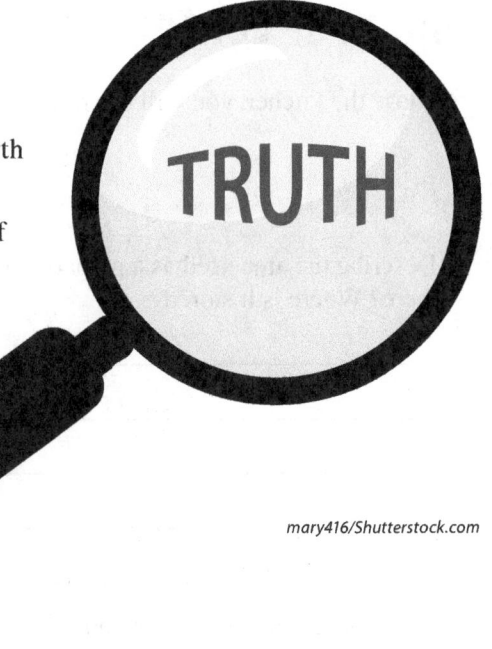

mary416/Shutterstock.com

Name _____ Date _____ Period _____

Activity D Lesson 5.3

Find Your Center

Choose the kitchen you will use to complete this activity and then answer the questions that follow. Choose one:

Home kitchen

Classroom kitchen

1. Describe the area used as a preparation and storage center. What appliance(s) is the center near? What is stored there? Where is it stored?

   _____
   _____
   _____
   _____
   _____

2. Describe the area used as a cooking and serving center. What appliance(s) is the center near? What is stored there? Where is it stored?

   _____
   _____
   _____
   _____
   _____
   _____

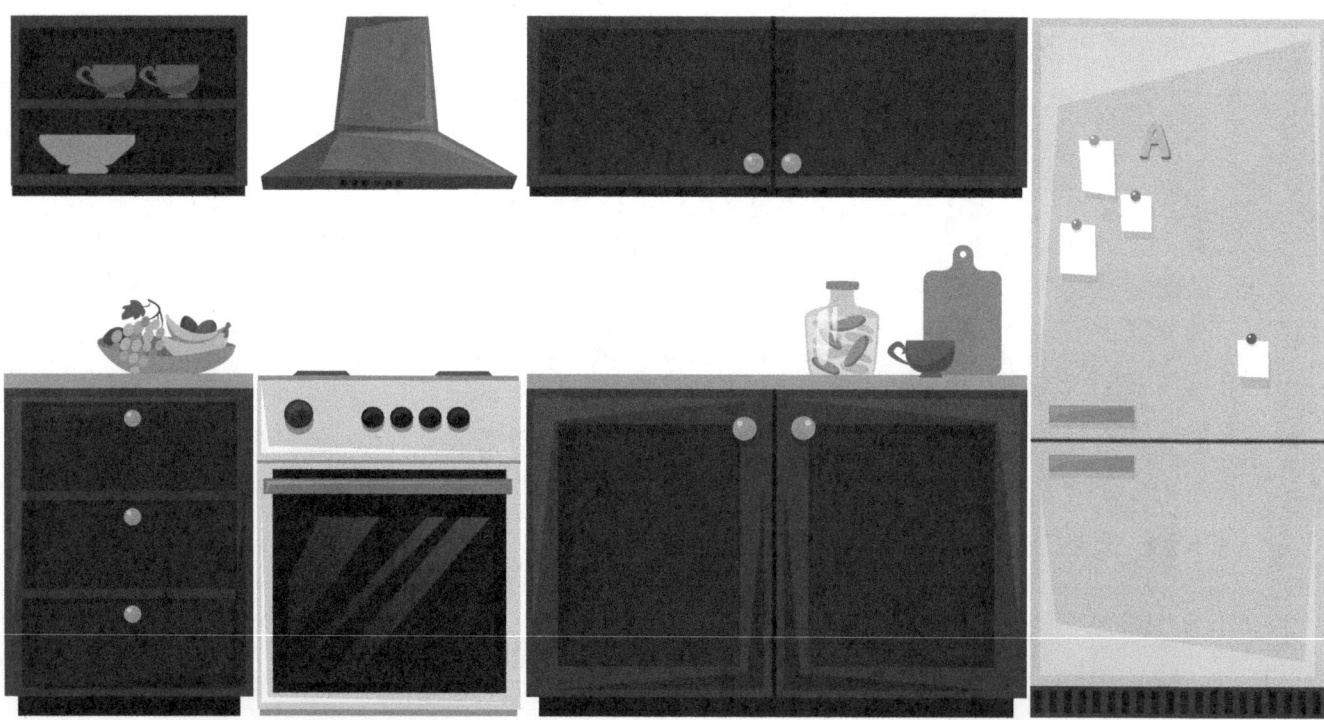

Tatiana Arestova/Shutterstock.com

(Continued)

Name _____ Date _____ Period _____

3. Describe the area used as a cleanup center. What appliance(s) is the center near? What is stored there? Where is it stored?

_____
_____
_____
_____
_____
_____

4. Describe the area used as an eating center. Where is it located?

_____
_____
_____
_____
_____
_____

5. Describe the area used as a planning and message center. What is stored there? Where is it stored?

_____
_____
_____
_____
_____
_____

6. Pick one of the centers you described above. What changes could be made to make the center work more effectively or efficiently?

Center: _____

_____
_____
_____
_____
_____
_____
_____
_____
_____
_____
_____

Name _____ Date _____ Period _____

Activity E   Chapter 5

New Terms Review

Read each definition and indicate which term is being described.

Definitions

1. _____ A large, costly machine used for everyday household tasks.
2. _____ A type of oven that cooks food with hot air.
3. _____ A type of oven that cooks food using superheated steam.
4. _____ A type of oven that cooks food by converting electricity into microwaves.
5. _____ A type of electromagnetic energy.
6. _____ A device that converts electricity into microwaves.
7. _____ A substance that changes between gas and liquid as it transfers heat out of a refrigerator.
8. _____ Area in the kitchen where a certain type of task is done and the equipment needed for the task is stored.
9. _____ The seller's guarantee that a product will perform as specified and will be replaced or repaired if it fails within a certain time.

Terms

A. magnetron
B. major appliance
C. microwave
D. microwave oven
E. refrigerant
F. steam oven
G. thermal oven
H. warranty
I. work center

Name _____ Date _____ Period _____

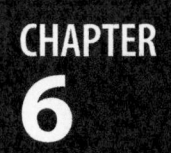 CHAPTER 6 — The Cook's Tools

Activity A   Lesson 6.1

Name That Tool

Place the correct term under each image. Use the terms from the word bank provided. Each term is used once.

Boning knife	Dry measuring cups	Metal spatula	Rubber spatula	Spoon
Can opener	Grater	Mixing bowl	Salad spinner	Strainer
Chef's knife	Kitchen fork	Paring knife	Scale	Tongs
Colander	Kitchen shears	Pastry blender	Slicer knife	Turner
Cookie cutter	Ladle	Pastry brush	Sifter	Utility knife
Cooling rack	Liquid measuring cup	Rolling pin	Slotted spoon	Vegetable peeler
Cutting board	Measuring spoons	Rotary beater	Spiral slicer	Whisk
Wire mesh sieve				

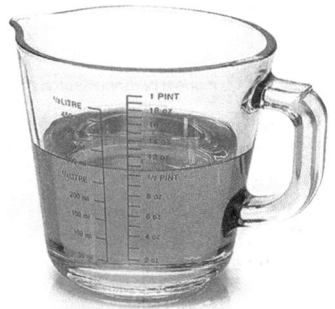
M. Unal Ozmen/Shutterstock.com

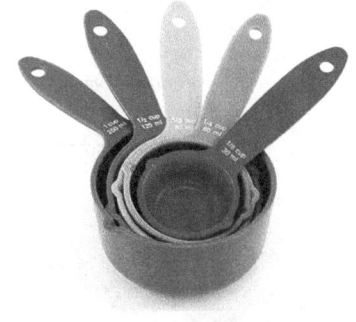
WhitePlaid/Shutterstock.com

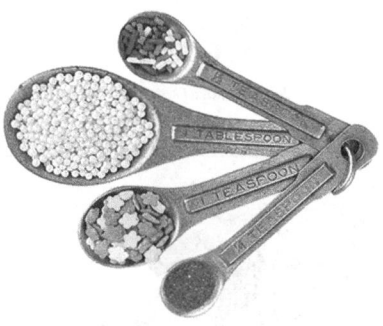
kasha_malasha/Shutterstock.com

1. _____ 2. _____ 3. _____

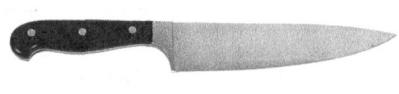

Africa Studio/Shutterstock.com   *Dron skm/Shutterstock.com*   *Matt Valentine/Shutterstock.com*

4. _____ 5. _____ 6. _____

(Continued)

Name _____ Date _____ Period _____

Dron skm/Shutterstock.com

karakedi35/Shutterstock.com

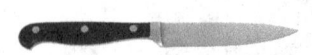
Dron skm/Shutterstock.com

7. _____ 8. _____ 9. _____

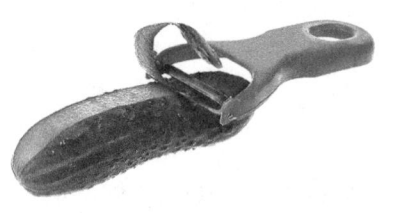
Goldution/Shutterstock.com

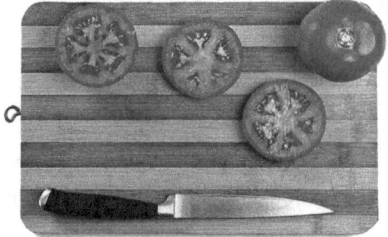
Yurchyks/Shutterstock.com

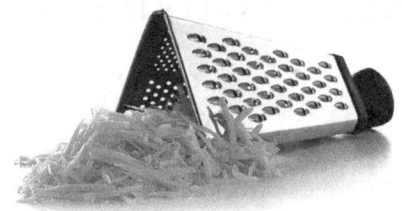
Africa Studio/Shutterstock.com

10. _____ 11. _____ 12. _____

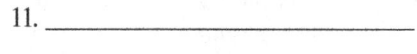
Serebryakova Ekaterina/Shutterstock.com

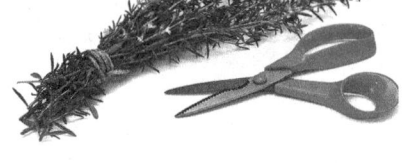
Andreja Donko/Shutterstock.com

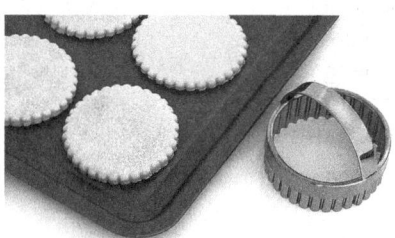
marilyn barbone/Shutterstock.com

13. _____ 14. _____ 15. _____

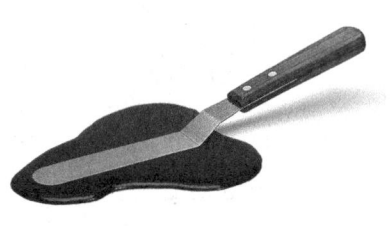
LSaloni/Shutterstock.com

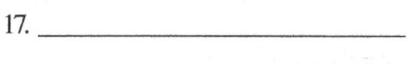
M. Unal Ozmen/Shutterstock.com

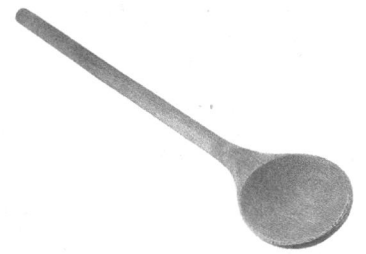
gmstockstudio/Shutterstock.com

16. _____ 17. _____ 18. _____

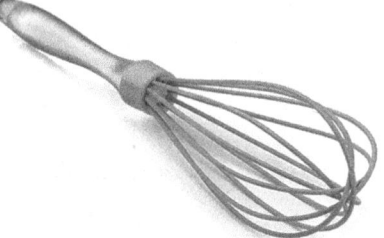
Coprid/Shutterstock.com

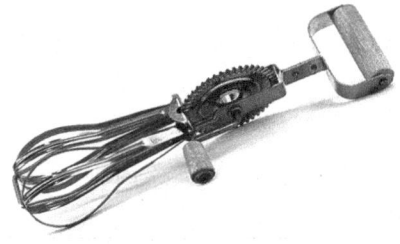
kavring/Shutterstock.com

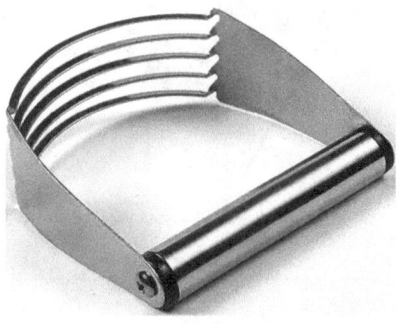
Brian McEntire/Shutterstock.com

19. _____ 20. _____ 21. _____

(Continued)

Name _____ Date _____ Period _____

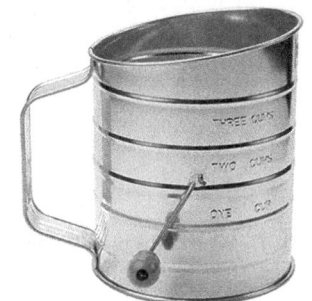
Danny Smythe/Shutterstock.com

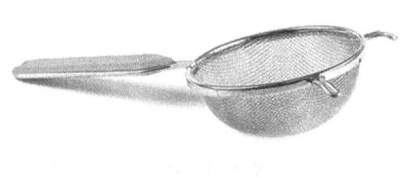
object ph/Shutterstock.com

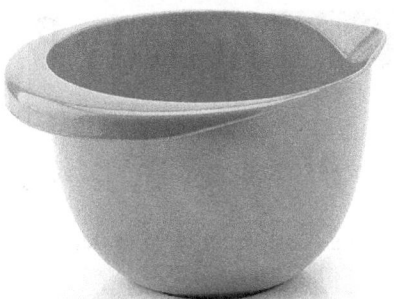
VictorH11/Shutterstock.com

22. _____

23. _____

24. _____

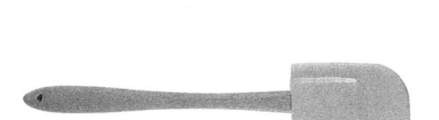
Naruedom Yaempongsa/Shutterstock.com

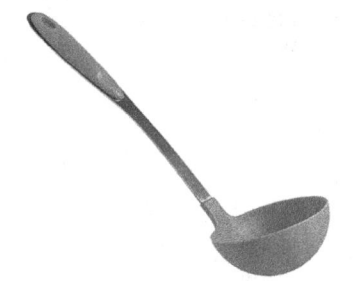
Oleksandr Nagaiets/Shutterstock.com

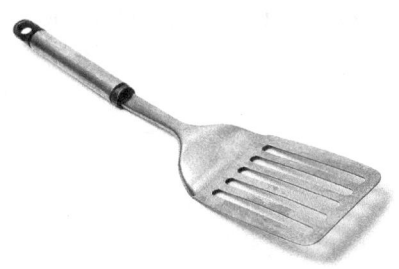
nito/Shutterstock.com

25. _____

26. _____

27. _____

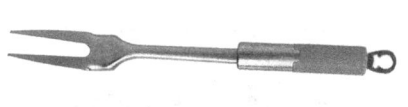
GeniusKp/Shutterstock.com

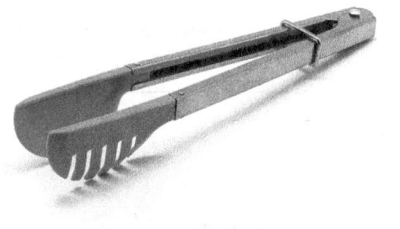
Mariontxa/Shutterstock.com

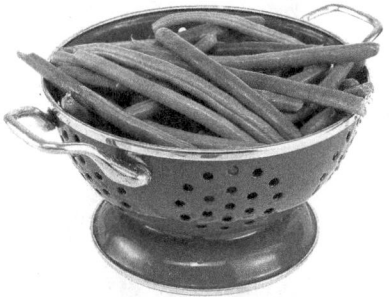
RoJo Images/Shutterstock.com

28. _____

29. _____

30. _____

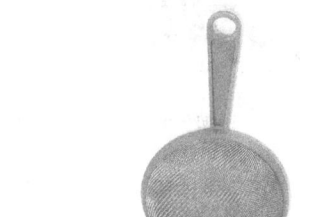
Vinte/Shutterstock.com

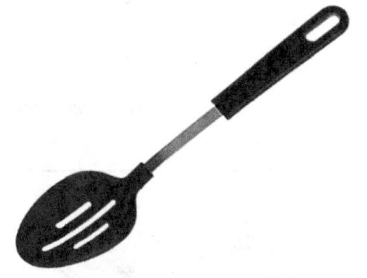
You Touch Pix of EuToch/Shutterstock.com

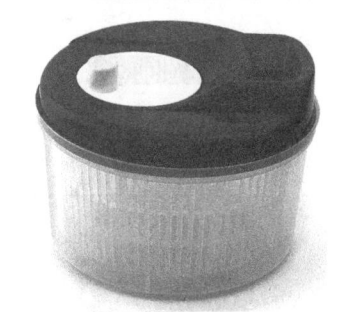
Vinte/Shutterstock.com

31. _____

32. _____

33. _____

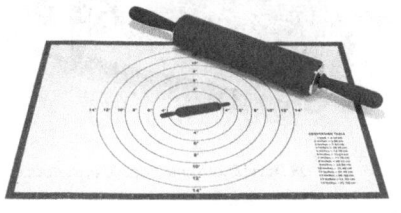
Michael Kraus/Shutterstock.com

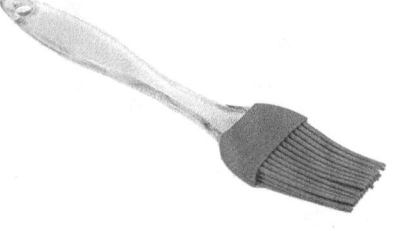
anmbph/Shutterstock.com

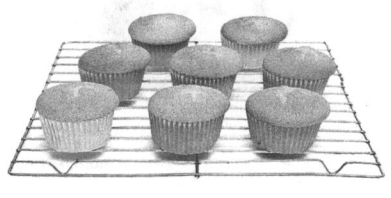
Crepesoles/Shutterstock.com

34. _____

35. _____

36. _____

Copyright Goodheart-Willcox Co., Inc.
May not be reproduced or posted to a publicly accessible website.

Chapter 6   The Cook's Tools   33

Name _____ Date _____ Period _____

 **Activity B Lesson 6.2**

Name That Appliance

Place the correct term under each image. Use the terms from the word bank provided. Each term is used once.

Blender	Electric skillet	Mixer	Roasting pan	Toaster
Casserole dish	Food processor	Muffin pan	Saucepan	Toaster oven
Coffeemaker	Griddle	Panini maker	Skillet	Tube pan
Cookie sheet	Immersion blender	Pie pan	Slow cooker	Wok
Double boiler	Loaf pan	Pot	Steamer	

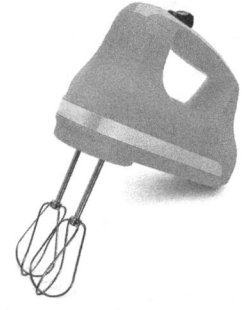
Iasha/Shutterstock.com

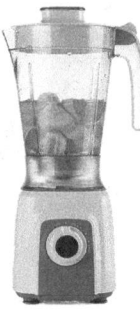
George Dolgikh/Shutterstock.com

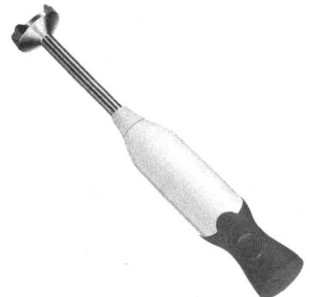
Zovteva/Shutterstock.com

1. _____   2. _____   3. _____

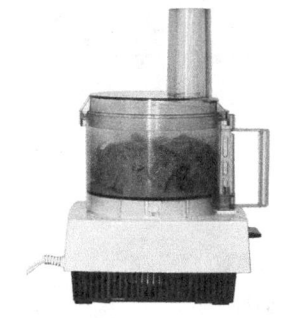
Le Do/Shutterstock.com

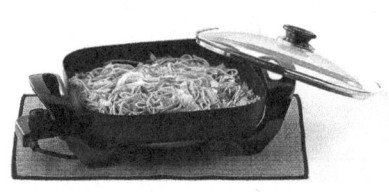
Venus Angel/Shutterstock.com

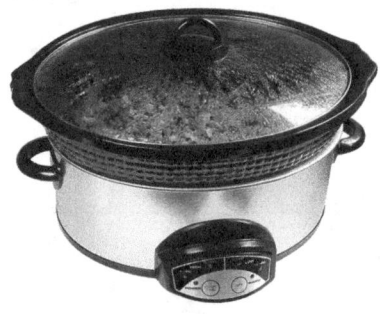
KellyNelson/Shutterstock.com

4. _____   5. _____   6. _____

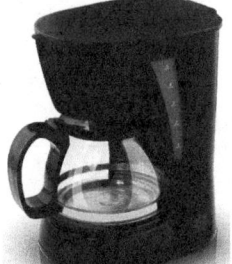
GzP_Design/Shutterstock.com

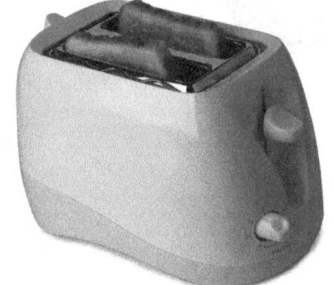
Dmitry Vinogradov/Shutterstock.com

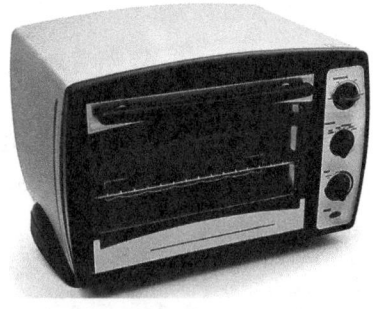
DR Travel Photo and Video/Shutterstock.com

7. _____   8. _____   9. _____

(Continued)

Name _____ Date _____ Period _____

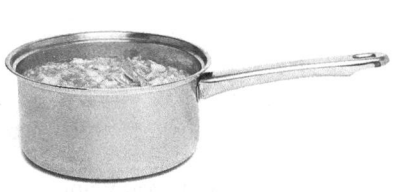
Crepesoles/Shutterstock.com

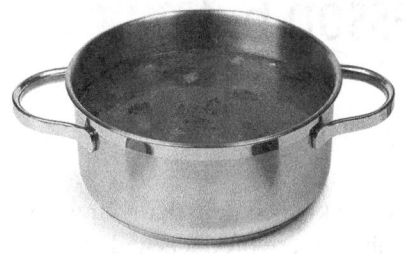
Timmary/Shutterstock.com

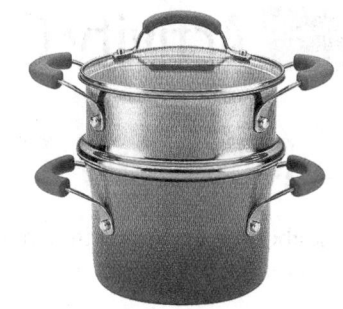
Beauty Creative/Shutterstock.com

10. _____ 11. _____ 12. _____

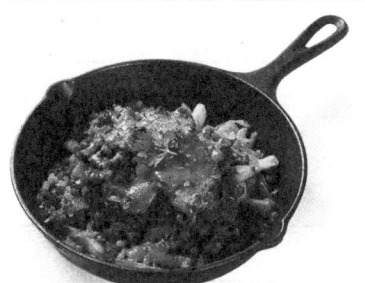
ben bryant/Shutterstock.com

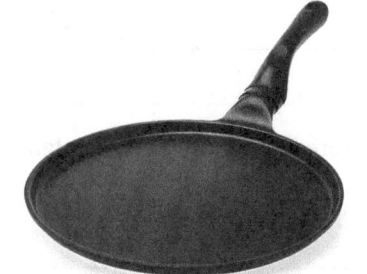
Olga Popova/Shutterstock.com

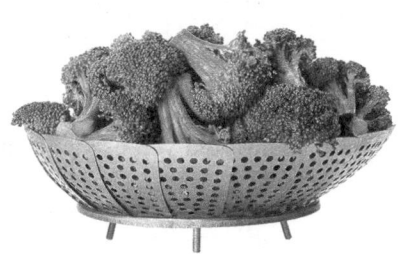
Cathleen A Clapper/Shutterstock.com

13. _____ 14. _____ 15. _____

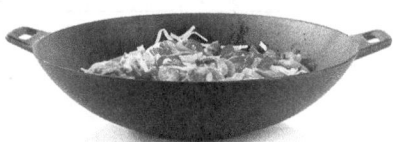
Africa Studio/Shutterstock.com

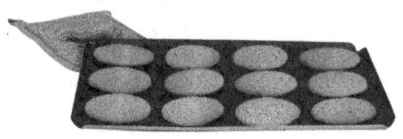
mikeledray/Shutterstock.com

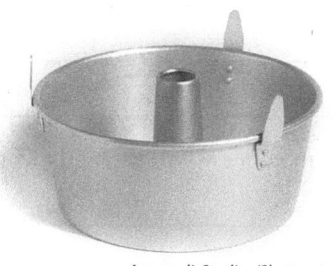
AnnapolisStudios/Shutterstock.com

16. _____ 17. _____ 18. _____

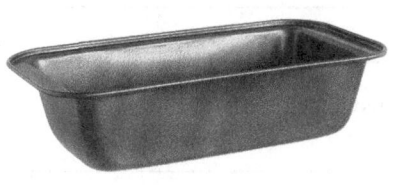
ratmaner/Shutterstock.com

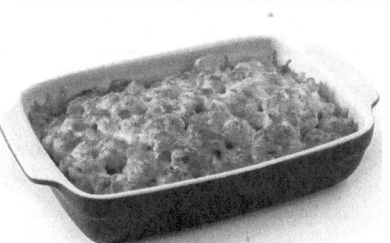
Poto69/Shutterstock.com

19. _____ 20. _____ 21. _____

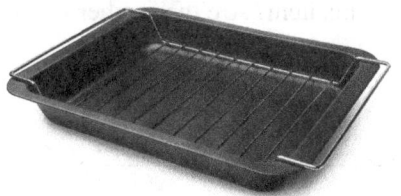
JeniFoto/Shutterstock.com

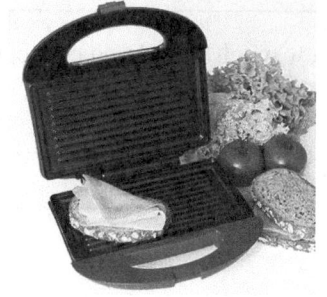
Olga Popova/Shutterstock.com

gcafotografia/Shutterstock.com

22. _____ 23. _____ 24. _____

Copyright Goodheart-Willcox Co., Inc.
May not be reproduced or posted to a publicly accessible website.

Chapter 6   The Cook's Tools   **35**

Name _____ Date _____ Period _____

Activity C Lesson 6.3

Should You Buy It?

Think about your home kitchen. Identify one kitchen item that you need and one kitchen item that you want. Research online or in stores to learn more about these products and then answer the question that follow.

Kitchen item you need: _____

1. Explain why you need this item.
   _____
   _____

2. How often would you use the item if it were in your kitchen? Explain your answer.
   _____
   _____

3. Is there a convenient place to store the item? If so, where? If not, will this affect how often you use the item?
   _____
   _____
   _____

4. Is the item easy to use and clean? Explain your answer.
   _____
   _____

5. Is it the right size to meet your family's needs? Explain your answer.
   _____
   _____

6. Is the item safe to use? Explain your answer.
   _____
   _____

7. Does this product have a warranty? Does this affect your purchase decision?
   _____

8. How much would you expect to pay for this item? Are there other less expensive models that would meet your needs?
   _____
   _____

(Continued)

Name _____ Date _____ Period _____

Kitchen item you want: _____

9. Explain why you want this item.
   _____
   _____

10. How often would you use the item if it were in your kitchen? Explain your answer.
    _____
    _____

11. Is there a convenient place to store the item? If so, where? If not, will this affect how often you use the item?
    _____
    _____
    _____

12. Is the item easy to use and clean? Explain your answer.
    _____
    _____

13. Is it the right size to meet your family's needs? Explain your answer.
    _____
    _____

14. Is the item safe to use? Explain your answer.
    _____
    _____

15. Does this product have a warranty? Does this affect your purchase decision?
    _____

16. How much would you expect to pay for this item? Are there other less expensive models that would meet your needs?
    _____
    _____

17. After answering the questions in this activity, have your thoughts changed about either the item that you need or the item that you want? Explain your answer.
    _____
    _____
    _____

Name _____ Date _____ Period _____

Activity D Chapter 6

New Terms Review

Read each definition and indicate which term is being described.

Definitions

1. _____ Having a sawtooth edge.
2. _____ Part of the knife blade that attaches to the knife handle.
3. _____ An action resulting from rotating an object that causes the object to move away from the center of rotation.
4. _____ Electrical tools that can be moved easily from one place to another.
5. _____ All the items used to serve and eat a meal.
6. _____ Serving containers that can hold more than a single serving.
7. _____ A slick coating applied to cookware and bakeware that prevents food from clinging and makes cleanup easier.

Terms

A. centrifugal force
B. hollowware
C. nonstick finish
D. serrated
E. small appliances
F. tableware
G. tang

Name _____ Date _____ Period _____

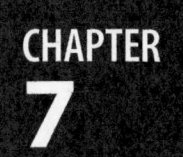

Play It Safe!

Activity A   Lesson 7.1

*Un*safe Stanley

Read the passage below. Determine which behaviors are unsafe. For every unsafe behavior, indicate the safe behavior that Stanley should have performed in the right-hand column. Include the number of the sentence/behavior that is being corrected.

Trueffelpix/Shutterstock.com

*Un*safe Stanley	Safe Stanley
(1) One day, Stanley decided to impress his friends by making home-cooked spaghetti with meat sauce for them. (2) In the kitchen, he got out a large pot and a saucepan. (3) He filled the pot nearly to the brim with water. (4) He placed the pot on the stove, put a lid on the pot, and turned the burner on high. (5) As he waited for the water to boil, he got the ground beef out of the refrigerator. (6) He unwrapped the raw meat and placed it on the cutting board while he gathered the rest of his ingredients. (7) The spices were stored at the top of the cabinet, so he climbed on the counter to reach them. (8) He then added the meat to the saucepan, placed it on the stove, turned the burner on high, and let the meat cook. (9) Next, Stanley placed an onion on the same cutting board and began cutting it with a chef's knife. (10) He had selected a dull knife because his knife skills are lacking and he reasoned that if the knife slipped, he would not hurt himself as badly.	

(*Continued*)

Name _____ Date _____ Period _____

Unsafe Stanley	Safe Stanley
(11) While cutting the onion, he thought he heard the water boiling over. (12) In his rush to check the water, he dropped the knife and tried to catch it. (13) He was unsuccessful and the knife fell to the floor. (14) When he checked the water, he lifted the lid straight up. (15) The water was not yet boiling, so he returned the lid, grabbed the knife off the floor, and continued to cut the onion. (16) Then he added the onion and seasonings to the beef. (17) He cooked the beef mixture until it was brown. (18) To finish the meat sauce, Stanley used the can opener to open the can of tomato sauce. (19) He stopped just before the lid was completely detached and bent the lid back so he could pour the sauce into the pan. (20) He brought the meat sauce to a simmer. (21) While the sauce was simmering, he added the pasta to the water. (22) When the pasta was cooked, he drained it using a colander, tossed it with the sauce, and placed it on a serving dish. (23) Pleased with his accomplishment, Stanley turned off the stove, threw his pot holder on the stovetop, and brought the meal out to his friends.	

Name _____ Date _____ Period _____

Activity B Lesson 7.2

Responding to Accidents

For each of the following scenarios, indicate the appropriate response.

Scenario	Response
Keisha cut herself while making carrot sticks for a snack.	
Robert spilled water on the floor while washing dishes and did not clean it up immediately. He later slipped on the wet floor and landed on his arm.	
Etaf received an electrical shock as she was trying to insert the damaged plug of a frayed electric cord into the wall outlet. She is lying on the floor a few feet from the plug and is unconscious.	
Santino was holding the pot holder incorrectly as he removed cookies from the oven. His finger touched the hot pan, and he received a burn. The burn is about the size of a dime.	
Maria was cleaning the kitchen while babysitting her little cousin. The phone rang and Maria went to answer the phone. On her return, she saw her cousin drinking some of the cleaning product she had been using.	
Your sister, Kaitlin, was eating a hot dog while playing video games. She had a mouthful of hot dog when she began cheering to celebrate the points she had scored. She began to choke on the hot dog.	

Name _____ Date _____ Period _____

Activity C Chapter 7

New Terms Review

Read each definition and indicate which term is being described.

Definitions

1. _____ A colorless, odorless, deadly gas.
2. _____ Treatment given immediately after an accident that helps to relieve pain and prevent further injury.
3. _____ A lifesaving method that includes forcing the victim's heart to pump blood and provides rescue breathing.
4. _____ A substance that reverses the effect of a poison.
5. _____ A maneuver that can save the life of a person who is choking.

Terms

A. abdominal thrust
B. antidote
C. carbon monoxide
D. cardiopulmonary resuscitation (CPR)
E. first aid

Name _____ Date _____ Period _____

CHAPTER 8
Keep It Clean!

Activity A Lesson 8.1

Recognizing the Enemy

For each cause of foodborne illness listed in the table, complete the sections with information from the text.

Pathogens			
Name	**Description**	**Common Source(s)**	**Example(s)**
Bacteria			
Viruses			
Parasites			
Molds			N/A
Toxins			

Copyright Goodheart-Willcox Co., Inc.
May not be reproduced or posted to a publicly accessible website.

Designua/Shutterstock.com

43

Name _____ Date _____ Period _____

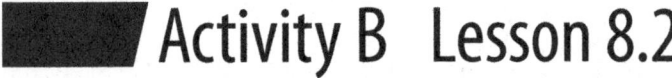 Activity B Lesson 8.2

Cleaning Poster Power

You have been hired by a textbook company to create a set of classroom posters to accompany Lesson 8.2, *Keeping Food Safe to Eat*. For each poster title, summarize the topic with four pieces of advice for cooks in your classroom.

Keep Yourself Clean!

1. _____
2. _____
3. _____
4. _____

Keep Your Kitchen Clean!

1. _____
2. _____
3. _____
4. _____

(Continued)

Name _____ Date _____ Period _____

Separate: Don't Cross-Contaminate!

1. _____
   _____
2. _____
   _____
3. _____
   _____
4. _____
   _____

Chill and Cook: Keep Food out of Danger Zone Temperatures!

1. _____
   _____
2. _____
   _____
3. _____
   _____
4. _____
   _____

Name _____ Date _____ Period _____

Activity C   Chapter 8

New Terms Review

Read each definition and indicate which term is being described.

Definitions

1. _____ Disease caused by a pathogen in food.
2. _____ An organism or substance that invades the body and damages its cells.
3. _____ Tiny organisms that are found everywhere, a few types can cause foodborne illness.
4. _____ Temperatures at which bacteria grow fastest; 40°F–140°F (5°C–60°C).
5. _____ Another word for poison.
6. _____ Spreading bacteria or other pathogens to a food from contaminated work surfaces, utensils, hands, or food.
7. _____ The use of methods that create a clean, healthy environment.

Terms

A. bacteria
B. cross-contamination
C. foodborne illness
D. pathogen
E. sanitation
F. temperature danger zone
G. toxin

Name _____ Date _____ Period _____

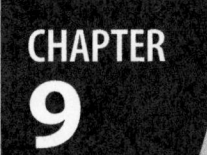

Recipes—Blueprints for Food

Activity A   Lesson 9.1

A Well-Written Recipe

Read the recipes that follow. Identify what components of a well-written recipe are missing in the spaces provided.

Recipe: Basic Crepes	
Ingredients	**Directions**
1 cup flour 2 eggs ½ cup milk ½ cup water ¼ teaspoon salt 2 tablespoons butter, melted	1. Whisk the flour and eggs together. Gradually add in the milk and water, stirring to combine. Add the salt and butter; beat until smooth. 2. Lightly grease the pan. Pour approximately ¼ cup of batter into the pan and cook over medium-high heat. Tilt the pan with a circular motion so the batter coats the surface evenly. 3. Cook the crepe for about 2 minutes, until the bottom is light brown. Loosen the edges, turn, and cook the other side. Serve hot.

1. What component(s) of a well-written recipe are missing from the basic crepe recipe above?

_____
_____
_____

Recipe: Quesadillas	
Ingredients	**Directions**
butter cheese, shredded flour tortillas salsa sour cream	1. Melt half of the butter in a large skillet. Place a tortilla in the skillet and fry one side, then remove it from the pan. Put the remaining butter in the pan, then place the unfried tortilla in the skillet. 2. Sprinkle cheese on top of the tortilla in the pan and top with the previously fried tortilla, browned side up. Press the tortillas together with a spatula and fry the quesadilla until the cheese is melted. 3. Remove the quesadilla from the pan and cut in wedges. Top with sour cream and/or salsa.

2. What component(s) of a well-written recipe are missing from the quesadilla recipe above?

_____
_____
_____

Copyright Goodheart-Willcox Co., Inc.
May not be reproduced or posted to a publicly accessible website.

Name _____ Date _____ Period _____

Activity B Lesson 9.1

Measuring Is off the Charts!

Techniques used to measure ingredients vary depending on the ingredient. Based on what you learned in Lesson 9.1, indicate the equipment and the technique you would use to measure each of the ingredients in the chart that follows. Then answer the question at the bottom of the page.

Ingredient	Equipment Needed	Description of Technique
Flour		
Brown sugar		
Shortening		
Butter		
Milk		

Can liquid and dry measuring cups be used interchangeably? Explain your answer.

_____

_____

Name _____ Date _____ Period _____

Activity C   Lesson 9.1

Am I Making Enough?

You have invited 11 friends for lunch. You want to serve tomato soup, but the recipe only yields 6 servings. Calculate the conversion factor you would use to increase the yield. Then multiply each ingredient amount by the conversion factor so the recipe will yield 12 servings.

What conversion factor will you use to adjust the yield for the recipe? Show your work below, then use the conversion factor to adjust the ingredient amounts in the table. (*Hint:* Servings Needed ÷ Servings Original Recipe Yields = Conversion Factor)

_____

Tomato Soup		
Ingredient Amounts to Yield 6 servings	**Multiply by Conversion Factor**	**Ingredient Amounts to Yield 12 servings**
1 tablespoon unsalted butter		unsalted butter
1 tablespoon olive oil		olive oil
1 onion, thinly sliced		onion, thinly sliced
2 garlic cloves, crushed		garlic cloves, crushed
2 28-ounce cans whole peeled tomatoes		28-ounce cans whole peeled tomatoes
1 cup water		water
1 tablespoon sugar		sugar
1 teaspoon salt		salt
to taste black pepper		black pepper
1 pinch red pepper flakes		red pepper flakes
¼ teaspoon celery seed		celery seed
¼ teaspoon dried oregano		dried oregano

Directions
1. Heat butter and olive oil in a large saucepan over medium-low heat. Add in onion and garlic and cook until onion is soft and translucent, about 5 minutes.
2. Add tomatoes, water, sugar, salt, pepper, red pepper flakes, celery seed, and oregano. Bring to a boil. Reduce heat, cover, and simmer for 15 minutes.
3. Remove from heat and puree with an immersion blender. Reheat soup if needed and serve.

Name _____ Date _____ Period _____

Activity D   Lesson 9.1

Working with Measurement Equivalents

Sometimes when recipe yields are adjusted up or down, the resulting ingredient amounts are not easily measured. For example, measuring 12 tablespoons of an ingredient is inconvenient and more likely to result in an error. This amount may be more easily measured using measurement equivalents. The measurement equivalent for 12 tablespoons is ¾ cup. Knowing how to use measurement equivalents is useful when adjusting recipe yields.

Practice using measurement equivalents as you complete the table that follows. In the third column, identify the measuring tool(s) you would use to measure the equivalent amount. (*Hint:* Lesson 6.1 discusses standard measures for measuring tools.)

Ingredient Amount	Measurement Equivalent	Measuring Tools Needed
6 teaspoons		
24 fluid ounces		
⅓ fluid ounce		
8 pints		
48 ounces		
16 tablespoons		
4 cups		
16 fluid ounces		
3 teaspoons		
32 fluid ounces		
6 tablespoons		

50   Adventures in Food and Nutrition Workbook

Name _____ Date _____ Period _____

Activity E Lesson 9.2

Organizing Terms

Organize the following terms by category.

bake	braise	cube	grate	panbroil	puree	shred	stew
barbecue	broil	cut in	grease	parboil	roast	sift	stir
baste	chill	deep-fry	grind	pare	sauté	simmer	stir-fry
beat	chop	drain	julienne	peel	scald	slice	toast
blanch	cool	fold	knead	poach	scrape	steam	whip
boil	cream	freeze	mince	preheat			

Category	Terms
Preparing to cook	
Removing skin	
Cutting	
Mixing	
Cooking with fat	
Cooking with liquids	
Cooking with dry heat	
Cooling	

Name _____ Date _____ Period _____

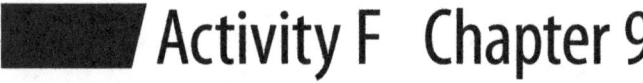 Activity F   Chapter 9

New (and Other) Terms Review

Read each definition and indicate which term is being described.

Definitions

1. _____ The space an ingredient occupies.
2. _____ The number and size of portions a recipe will make.
3. _____ Shortened form of a word.
4. _____ A food used to prepare a dish.
5. _____ The measure of how heavy an ingredient should be.
6. _____ The desirable color found on a food's surface as a result of many dry-heat cooking methods.
7. _____ A list of foods and directions for preparing a dish.

Terms

A. abbreviation
B. browning
C. ingredient
D. recipe
E. volume
F. weight
G. yield

Name _____ Date _____ Period _____

What's on the Menu?

Activity A   Lesson 10.1

A Blast with Brunch

Mother's Day is fast approaching and you have decided to use skills learned in Family and Consumer Sciences class to plan a Mother's Day Brunch for your family. You picked brunch because the menu can include both breakfast and lunch items. Indicate what you will be serving in the menu that follows. Be sure to include beverages.

Brunch Menu

PON-PON/Shutterstock.com

(Continued)

Name _____ Date _____ Period _____

Explain how your menu addresses each of the following factors that make a meal appealing.

1. Colors

   _____
   _____
   _____
   _____

2. Shapes and Sizes

   _____
   _____
   _____
   _____

3. Textures

   _____
   _____
   _____
   _____

4. Temperatures

   _____
   _____
   _____
   _____

5. Cooking Methods

   _____
   _____
   _____
   _____

6. Flavors

   _____
   _____
   _____
   _____

Name _____ Date _____ Period _____

Activity B Lesson 10.2

Convenience Scavenger Hunt

Explore the cabinets and refrigerator at home or in your school kitchen as directed by your teacher. Find five food items that you believe are convenience foods. For each food item, indicate if it is *Ready to Eat*, *Partially Prepared*, *Minimally Processed*, or *Highly Processed*. (More than one may apply to some food items.)

Food Item	Ready to Eat	Partially Prepared	Minimally Processed	Highly Processed

What is the benefit of using these convenience foods? What are the drawbacks? Explain your answers.

_____

_____

_____

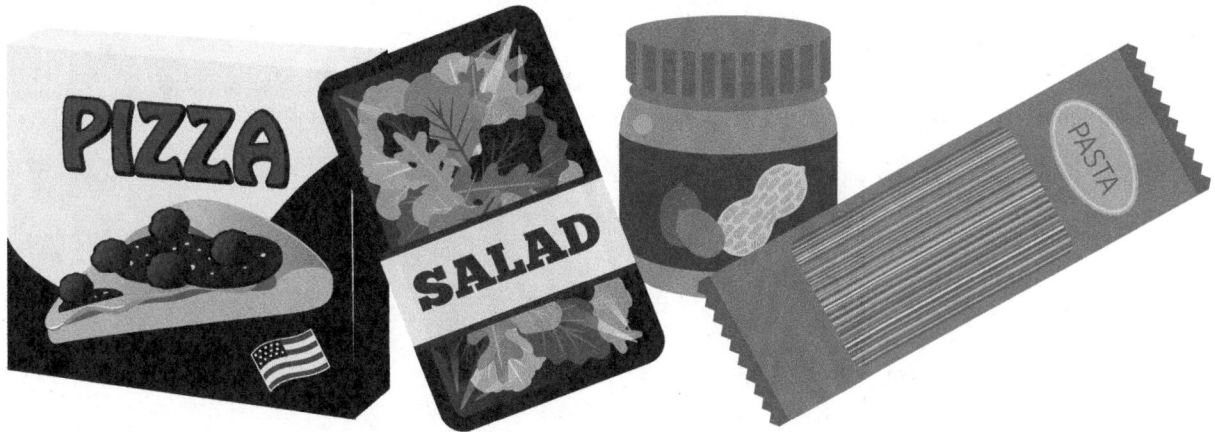

(peanut butter) lukpedclub/Shutterstock.com; (salad) Tarikdiz/Shutterstock.com; (pizza) Altagracia Art/Shutterstock.com; (pasta) KittyVector/Shutterstock.com

Name _____ Date _____ Period _____

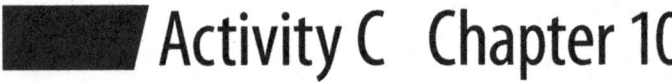 Activity C Chapter 10

New Terms Review

Read each definition and indicate which term is being described.

Definitions

1. _____ Ways and means, such as time and money, available to complete a task.
2. _____ Food that requires little or no preparation before eating.
3. _____ Food that retains most of the physical and nutritional qualities that it had at harvest.
4. _____ Food that undergoes complex preparation procedures to lengthen shelf life and shorten preparation time; sugar, sodium, and fat are often added to improve flavor or preserve the shelf life of these foods.
5. _____ A decoration you can eat that adds color to meals.

Terms

A. convenience food
B. garnish
C. highly processed food
D. minimally processed food
E. resources

Name _____ Date _____ Period _____

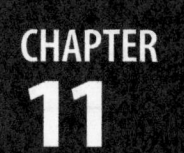

Smart Shopping

Activity A Lesson 11.1

Where Should They Shop?

For each of the following scenarios, decide whether the person should shop at a farmers market, supermarket, neighborhood grocery store, discount food store, specialty shop, food cooperative, or convenience store. (More than one answer may be applicable.) Justify your answer.

Scenario 1
Aniya is planning a small evening get together to meet her boyfriend's parents for the first time. She wants to impress them, but she is not going to cook a meal. She wants to find an array of fine cheeses, cured meats, fancy crackers, and other gourmet finger foods.

1. Where should Aniya shop? Justify your answer.

   _____
   _____

Scenario 2
Jake is a busy, single father of three school-age children. He has very little food left in the house. He needs to do food shopping for a wide variety of food items that can be used for all meals and snacks for him and his children for the whole week.

2. Where should Jake shop? Justify your answer.

   _____
   _____

3. List two tips to help Jake prepare for his shopping trip that will save him time, energy, and money.

   _____
   _____

Scenario 3
Marlen has a craving for her favorite meal. As she is leaving work, she decides she wants to make the meal, but she is missing a few key ingredients. Marlen will need to pick up the ingredients she needs on the way home.

4. Where should Marlen shop? Justify your answer.

   _____
   _____

(Continued)

Copyright Goodheart-Willcox Co., Inc.
May not be reproduced or posted to a publicly accessible website.

Name _____ Date _____ Period _____

Scenario 4
Santiago is getting ready to leave work when he receives a text from his daughter saying that they need milk. He plans to pick it up on his way home and does not want to go far out of his way.

5. Where should Santiago shop? Justify your answer.

_____
_____

Scenario 5
Maria is a 5th grade teacher and promised her class a reward for good behavior. She plans on picking up some ready-to-eat snack items such as doughnuts, chips, and cookies on her way to school to feed the class.

6. Where should Maria shop? Justify your answer.

_____
_____

Scenario 6
Jamal firmly believes in shopping local and supporting local agriculture. He does the majority of his shopping for paper products and other items that have a long shelf life at a discount food store. However, he likes to have fresh fruits and vegetables on hand to cook with on a daily basis.

7. Where should Jamal shop? Justify your answer.

_____
_____

Scenario 7
Stephanie has a growing family and they use a lot of food and paper products. Therefore, she likes to buy in bulk and is very conscious of saving money. She only likes to shop once a month because of her family's busy schedule.

8. Where should Stephanie shop? Justify your answer.

_____
_____

9. List two tips to help Stephanie prepare for her shopping trip that will save her time, energy, and money.

_____
_____

Name _____ Date _____ Period _____

Activity B Lesson 11.2

A Smart Shopper Sidekick

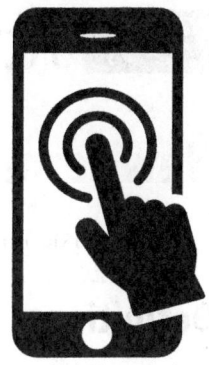

sommthink/Shutterstock.com

You have been hired by a consumer advocacy group to create an app to help people make smart decisions when shopping. The app is called the *Smart Shopper Sidekick*. Brainstorm four features that the app would have to help shoppers make smart decisions in the supermarket. Be creative! Justify why each feature is important to include in the app.

1. Feature name: _____

   What does the feature do?
   _____

   How does the feature help shoppers make smart shopping decisions?
   _____
   _____
   _____

2. Feature name: _____

   What does the feature do?
   _____

   How does the feature help shoppers make smart shopping decisions?
   _____
   _____
   _____

3. Feature name: _____

   What does the feature do?
   _____

   How does the feature help shoppers make smart shopping decisions?
   _____
   _____
   _____

4. Feature name: _____

   What does the feature do?
   _____

   How does the feature help shoppers make smart shopping decisions?
   _____
   _____
   _____

Name _____ Date _____ Period _____

Activity C Chapter 11

New Terms Review

Read each definition and indicate which term is being described.

Definitions

1. _____ A product made by a well-known company; the company's name appears on the packaging.
2. _____ Crops grown on farmland that has not been treated with human-made pesticides or weed killers or fertilized with sewage sludge; includes meats from farm animals that received no drugs or hormones to speed their growth rate.
3. _____ Food that can be safely stored at room temperature and stays fresh for a long time.
4. _____ The cost per unit of an item.
5. _____ A product that has no brand; often the least expensive.
6. _____ Any substance added to foods.
7. _____ A product made for a supermarket chain; the store's name may or may not appear on the packaging.
8. _____ Making an unplanned purchase.
9. _____ A substance that your body identifies as an invader, which causes an immune response.
10. _____ A system of labeling foods with dates to help you decide which package to buy and which to use first.
11. _____ A series of black lines, bars, and numbers printed on food labels used to identify the product, its manufacturer, size, style or form, and current price.
12. _____ Comparing prices of different brands, forms, and sizes of the same item.
13. _____ Food that spoils in a few days.

Terms

A. allergen
B. comparison shopping
C. food additive
D. generic product
E. impulse buying
F. name brand
G. open dating
H. organic food
I. perishable food
J. shelf-stable food
K. store brand
L. unit price
M. universal product code (UPC)

Name _____ Date _____ Period _____

CHAPTER 12 Ready, Set, Cook!

Activity A   Lesson 12.1

Team Time Checklist

Menu

Recall your favorite meal to prepare and record it in the box labeled "Menu." Then create a checklist of all the tasks that must be done to prepare, clean up, and evaluate the meal.

✓ _____
✓ _____
✓ _____
✓ _____
✓ _____
✓ _____
✓ _____
✓ _____
✓ _____
✓ _____
✓ _____
✓ _____
✓ _____
✓ _____
✓ _____
✓ _____
✓ _____
✓ _____
✓ _____
✓ _____
✓ _____
✓ _____
✓ _____
✓ _____
✓ _____
✓ _____
✓ _____

Name _____ Date _____ Period _____

Activity B Lesson 12.2

Plan a Party

Imagine a special occasion that you want to celebrate and then answer the questions that follow to plan a party. Be sure to use terminology from the chapter.

1. What is the special occasion your party is celebrating?
   _____
   _____

2. How much money will you budget for the party?
   _____

3. How many people will you invite?
   _____

4. Where will the party be held?
   _____
   _____

5. What type of food will you serve?
   _____
   _____

6. How will you set the table and serve the food?
   _____
   _____
   _____

7. What type of entertainment will you have?
   _____
   _____
   _____

8. What type of decorations will you use?
   _____
   _____
   _____

9. What type of invitations will you send?
   _____
   _____

(Continued)

Name _____ Date _____ Period _____

10. What actions will you take as host to ensure your guests have a good time?
_____
_____
_____

11. What is your plan for cleaning up when the party is over?
_____
_____
_____

12. Describe an event or a party you have attended which was not well planned. Identify the aspect(s) that were poorly planned. What was the impact on the party and guests? What could have been done differently?
_____
_____
_____
_____
_____
_____
_____
_____
_____
_____

davooda/Shutterstock.com

Name _____ Date _____ Period _____

Activity C   Chapter 12

New (and Other) Terms Review

Read each definition and indicate which term is being described.

Definitions

1. _____ An abbreviation written on invitations that means "please reply."
2. _____ A serving style in which foods are placed on each person's plate in the kitchen and taken to the table.
3. _____ A plan that lists the time needed to prepare a meal, eat, and clean up.
4. _____ A serving style in which meals are served in courses.
5. _____ The main dish course.
6. _____ To perform two or more tasks at the same time.
7. _____ All the dinnerware, flatware, glassware, and table linen used by one person.
8. _____ A serving style in which each food is placed in a serving dish along with a serving utensil and then placed on a serving table.
9. _____ A serving style in which all foods are placed in serving dishes and placed on the table; each person serves his or her own plate and then passes the serving dish to the next person.
10. _____ The space needed for one place setting.

Terms

A. blue-plate style
B. buffet style
C. cover
D. entrée course
E. family style
F. formal style
G. multitask
H. place setting
I. RSVP
J. work schedule

Name _____ Date _____ Period _____

CHAPTER 13 — Eating on the Go

Activity A   Lesson 13.1

Idea Clouds

Using what you learned in Lesson 13.1, identify four ideas that would make healthy eating on the go easier. Ideas should include tasks that could be performed in advance so that healthy food options are ready to grab and go!

Copyright Goodheart-Willcox Co., Inc.
May not be reproduced or posted to a publicly accessible website.

Name _____ Date _____ Period _____

Activity B Lesson 13.1

Pizza Progress

Design your perfect, healthier pizza. In the first column, list the ingredients on pizza you typically eat. In the second column, indicate healthier alternative ingredients. Next time you make pizza, try making your healthier option and make progress toward a healthier eating plan!

Ingredient Category	Typical Pizza Ingredients	Healthier Pizza Ingredients
Crust		
Sauce		
Toppings		
Finishing Touches		

Name _____ Date _____ Period _____

Activity C Lesson 13.2

Your Lunch-on-the-Go Plan

It is your job to prepare your school lunches. In this activity, you will plan, prepare, and package healthy lunches for the week. For each day, plan a different packed lunch that is balanced and has variety. Describe the foods you will include and how you will package them.

Day	Food Items	Packaging
Monday		
Tuesday		
Wednesday		
Thursday		
Friday		

Name _____ Date _____ Period _____

Activity D   Lesson 13.2

Tips and Tips

Answer the questions in the space provided.

Scenario

You and your friend John are going to a new restaurant in town. John has never eaten at a full-service restaurant and he is not sure what to expect. He is unsure about ordering food, paying the check, and the proper manners to use. In addition, John has been trying to make healthier food choices and is afraid the temptation to make poor food choices will be too great.

1. What are four tips for eating at restaurants that would help John feel at ease?

   _____
   _____
   _____
   _____
   _____
   _____
   _____
   _____

2. What are two suggestions for John to help him select healthy options at the restaurant?

   _____
   _____
   _____

3. The bill arrives at the end of the meal. The service was excellent. The bill was $72.48 and John wants to leave a 20% tip. Calculate the tip. Show your work.

   _____
   _____

Mickicev Atelje/Shutterstock.com

68   Adventures in Food and Nutrition Workbook

Copyright Goodheart-Willcox Co., Inc.
May not be reproduced or posted to a publicly accessible website.

Name _____ Date _____ Period _____

CHAPTER 14 — Fabulous Fruits

Activity A   Lesson 14.1

Fruit Fact or Falsehood?

Indicate whether each of the following statements about fruit is true or false. If the statement is false, restate it to make the statement true in the space provided.

1. _____ Fruit contains the plant's seeds.
   _____

2. _____ All fruits, except avocados and coconuts, are low in fat and calories.
   _____

3. _____ Fruit is a poor source of phytonutrients.
   _____

4. _____ Fruit juice concentrates are very low in sugar and high in nutrients.
   _____

5. _____ Eat different colored fruits to get a variety of phytonutrients.
   _____

6. _____ Drupes that are dark yellow or orange on the inside are rich in vitamin D.
   _____

7. _____ The best citrus fruits are firm and heavy.
   _____

8. _____ Berries stop ripening once they are picked.
   _____

9. _____ A ripe melon makes a solid sound when tapped gently.
   _____

10. _____ Avocados and plantains are tropical fruits.
    _____

Name _____ Date _____ Period _____

Activity B Lesson 14.1

Picture It!

There are six types of fruit: drupe, pome, citrus, melon, berry, and tropical. In the space below each image, indicate what type each fruit is. Some types will be used more than once.

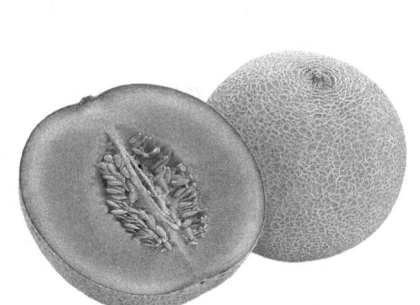
bergamont/Shutterstock.com

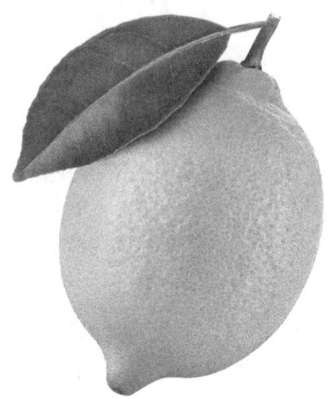
Maks Narodenko/Shutterstock.com

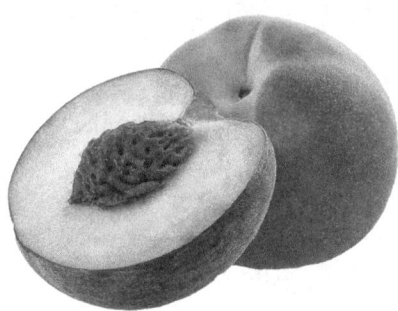
Viktar Malyshchyts/Shutterstock.com

1. _____ 2. _____ 3. _____

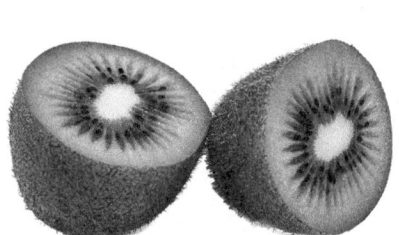
BestForBest/Shutterstock.com

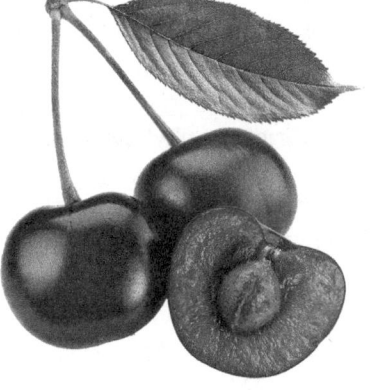
Valentyn Volkov/Shutterstock.com

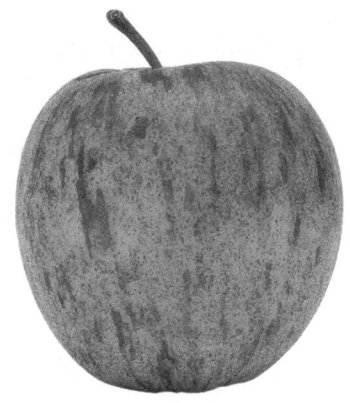
akepong srichaichana/Shutterstock.com

4. _____ 5. _____ 6. _____

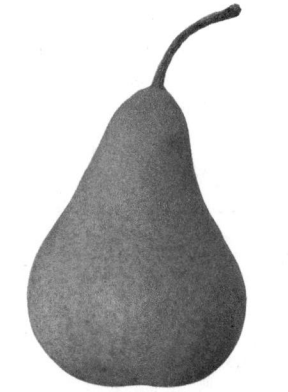
Bronwyn Photo/Shutterstock.com

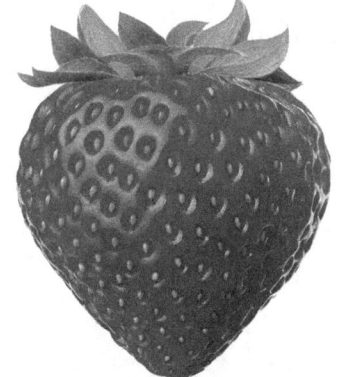
Valentina Razumova/Shutterstock.com

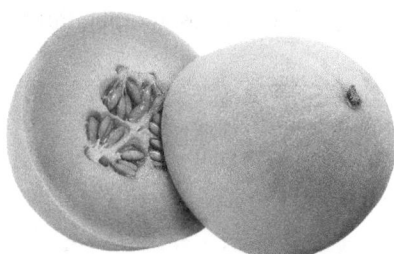
photosync/Shutterstock.com

7. _____ 8. _____ 9. _____

Name _____ Date _____ Period _____

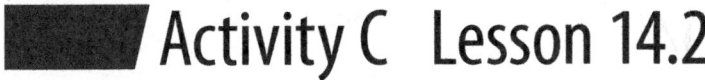 Activity C Lesson 14.2

Peachy Keen!

Respond to the following scenario with advice based on chapter content.

> **Scenario**
> Your Aunt Chaniece does not have great cooking skills. She recently moved to Georgia, and her new neighbors left a case of peaches on her doorstep as a welcome gift. She cannot possibly use all of the peaches before they go bad, so she wants to store some for future use and cook the rest. Remembering that you are a Family and Consumer Sciences student, your Aunt Chaniece asks you for advice.

Dear Aunt Chaniece,

_____
_____
_____
_____
_____
_____
_____
_____
_____
_____
_____
_____
_____
_____
_____
_____
_____
_____
_____
_____
_____
_____
_____
_____

Name _____ Date _____ Period _____

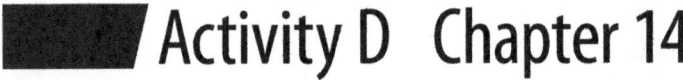 Activity D Chapter 14

New Terms Review

Read each definition and indicate which term is being described.

Definitions

1. ____ A type of fruit that has leathery skin, many segments filled with juicy pellets, and grows on trees.
2. ____ Fresh fruits and vegetables.
3. ____ A type of fruit with a core that contains seeds and grows on trees.
4. ____ A small, juicy fruit that contains many tiny seeds.
5. ____ A type of fruit that grows only in warm, sunny climates.
6. ____ A type of fruit that has one large pit or seed and grows on trees.
7. ____ A large, moist fruit that grows on a vine and contains seeds; has thick skin that may be smooth or rough.

Terms

A. berry
B. citrus fruit
C. drupe
D. melon
E. pome
F. produce
G. tropical fruit

Name _____ Date _____ Period _____

Versatile Vegetables

Activity A Lesson 15.1

Well Versed in Vegetables

In the middle column, provide one example of each type of vegetable. In the last column, identify characteristics to look for when selecting this type of vegetable.

Type	Example	Characteristics
Root Vegetables		
Tubers		
Bulb Vegetables		
Stalk Vegetables		
Leaf Vegetables		
Flower Vegetables		
Fruit Vegetables		
Seed Vegetables		

Copyright Goodheart-Willcox Co., Inc.
May not be reproduced or posted to a publicly accessible website.

Name _____ Date _____ Period _____

Activity B Lesson 15.2

Vegetable Memes

Turn the images that follow into memes by creating a clever caption or catchphrase for each. The caption should help you to remember content from the lesson by incorporating facts presented in the reading.

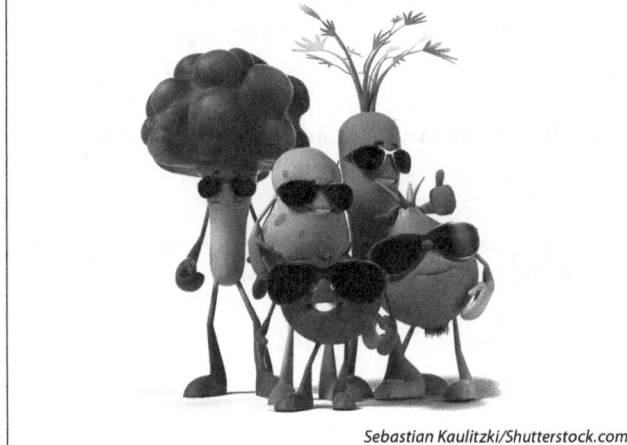
Sebastian Kaulitzki/Shutterstock.com

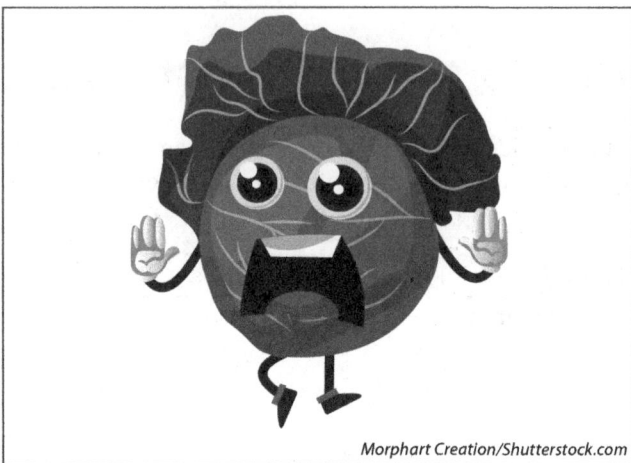
Morphart Creation/Shutterstock.com

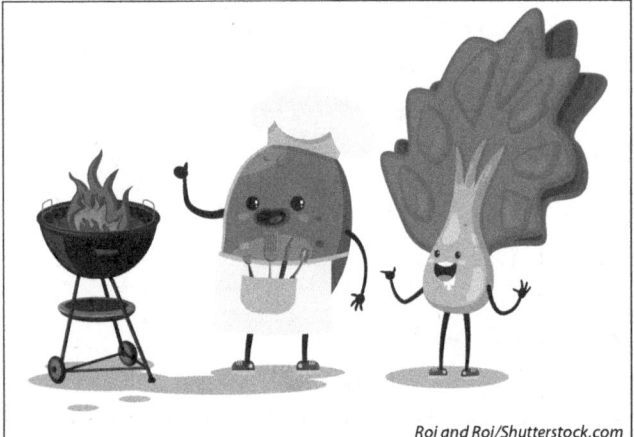
Roi and Roi/Shutterstock.com

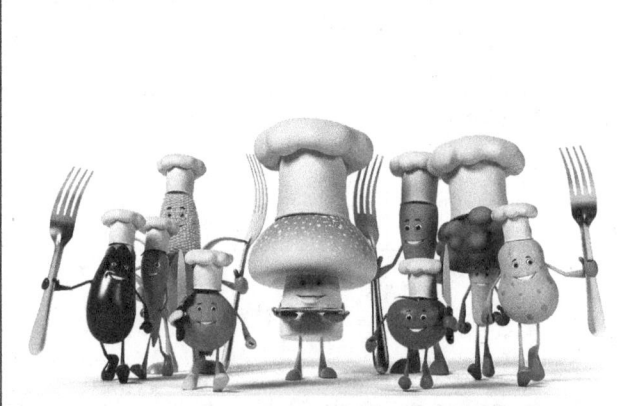
Sebastian Kaulitzki/Shutterstock.com

(Continued)

74 Adventures in Food and Nutrition Workbook

Name _____ Date _____ Period _____

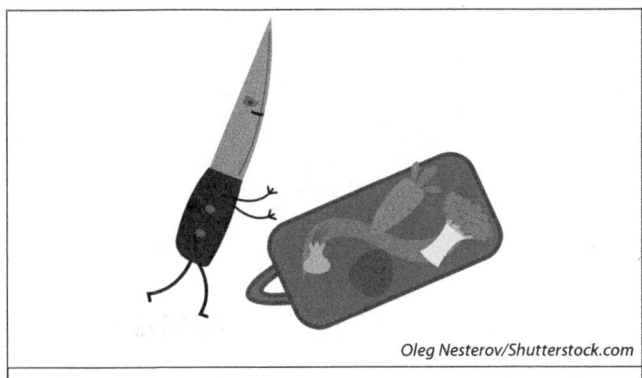
Oleg Nesterov/Shutterstock.com

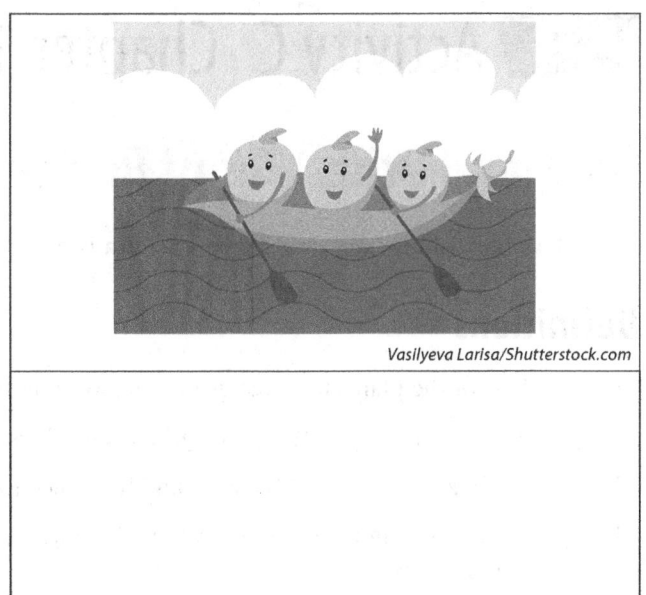
Vasilyeva Larisa/Shutterstock.com

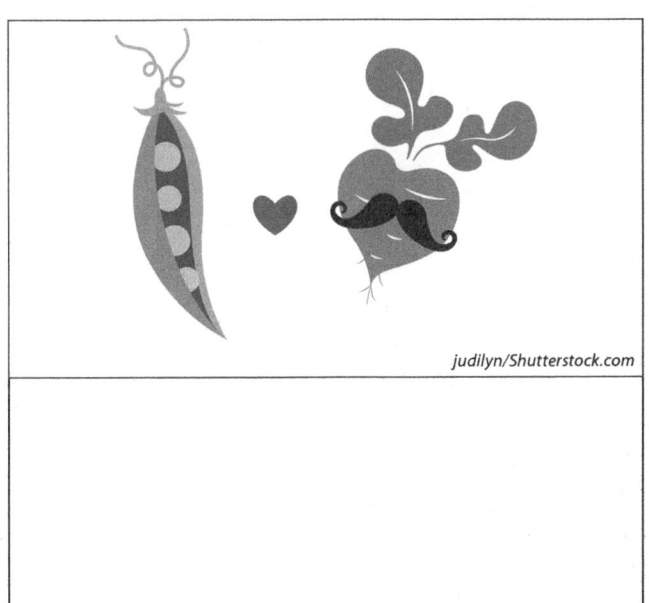
judilyn/Shutterstock.com

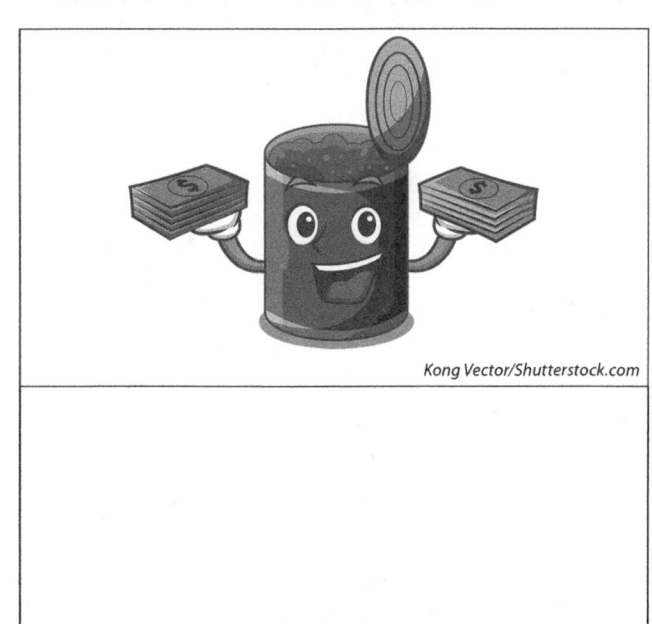
Kong Vector/Shutterstock.com

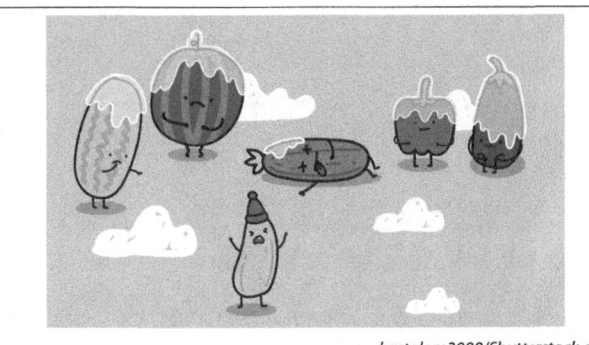

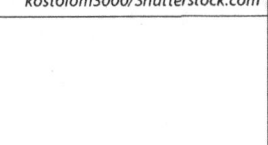
kostolom3000/Shutterstock.com

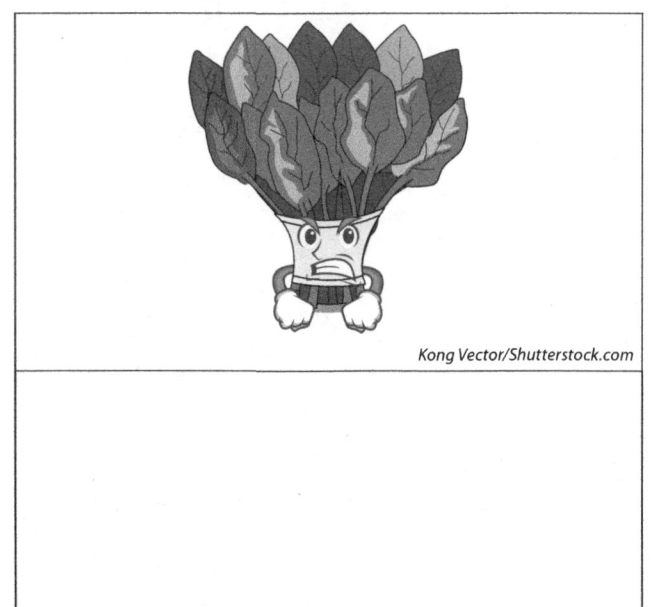
Kong Vector/Shutterstock.com

Copyright Goodheart-Willcox Co., Inc.
May not be reproduced or posted to a publicly accessible website.

Chapter 15 Versatile Vegetables 75

Name _____ Date _____ Period _____

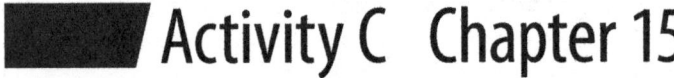 Activity C Chapter 15

New (and Other) Terms Review

Read each definition and indicate which term is being described.

Definitions

1. ____ Part of the plant stem that grows underground and swells to store food.
2. ____ The green pigment that gives green vegetables their color.
3. ____ An ingredient that adds flavor and fragrance to food.
4. ____ An orange pigment found in vegetables and fruits that can be converted to vitamin A in the body.
5. ____ A short, rounded bud that grows underground and stores food for the plant.

Terms

A. beta-carotene
B. bulb
C. chlorophyll
D. seasoner
E. tuber

Name ______________________ Date ______________ Period __________

CHAPTER 16

Salad Success

Activity A Lesson 16.1

aficons/Shutterstock.com

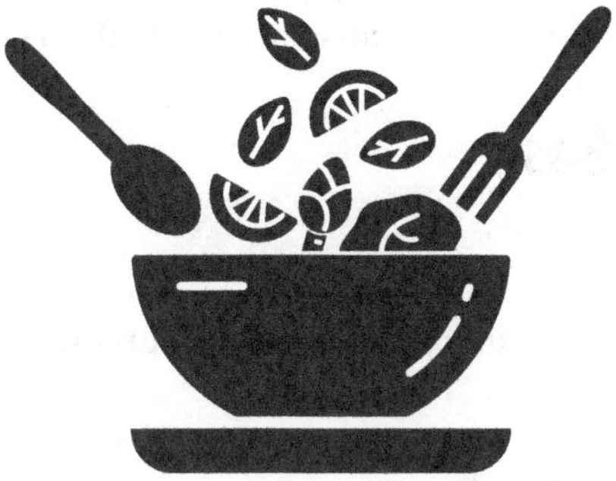

Salad Myth Busters

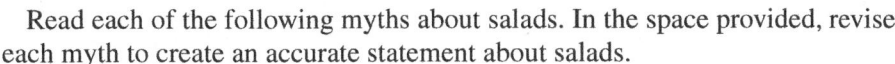

Read each of the following myths about salads. In the space provided, revise each myth to create an accurate statement about salads.

Myth #1: Salads supply few nutrients.

Myth #2: Vegetables are the only ingredient used to make salads.

Myth #3: Salads are always served at the beginning of a meal.

Myth #4: Congealed (gelatin) salads are always sweet and served for dessert.

Myth #5: Salad garnishes are added only for visual interest and should not be eaten.

Myth #6: Salad dressings should always be added to the salad a few hours before the salad is served to give flavors time to blend.

Name _____ Date _____ Period _____

Activity B Lesson 16.2

Your Ultimate Salad

In this activity, you will describe the base, body, garnish, and dressing that make up your "ultimate salad" and how those ingredients are prepared. Then, you will evaluate your salad by answering the questions that follow.

Base

_____

What ingredient(s) makes up the base?
_____

Why did you select this base?
_____
_____

How will you prepare the ingredient(s) for the base?
_____
_____

Body

_____

What ingredient(s) makes up the body?
_____

Why did you select this body?
_____
_____

How will you prepare the ingredient(s) for the body?
_____
_____

Garnish

_____

What ingredient(s) makes up the garnish?
_____

(Continued)

Name _____ Date _____ Period _____

Why did you select this garnish?
_____
_____

How will you prepare the ingredient(s) for the garnish?
_____
_____

Salad Dressing

_____

What type of salad dressing is this?
_____

What ingredient(s) makes up the salad dressing?
_____

Why did you select this salad dressing?
_____
_____

How will you prepare this dressing?
_____
_____

Evaluate

1. Is your "ultimate salad" nutrient rich? Explain your answer.
   _____
   _____

2. What ingredient(s) could you change or add to make your "ultimate salad" healthier? Explain your answer.
   _____
   _____

3. Is your "ultimate salad" appealing? Explain your answer.
   _____
   _____

4. Would you eat your "ultimate salad"? Explain your answer.
   _____
   _____

Name _____ Date _____ Period _____

Activity C   Chapter 16

New Terms Review

Read each definition and indicate which term is being described.

Definitions

1. ____ A gelling agent made from red algae; when mixed with liquid, it forms a firm, jelly-like consistency.

2. ____ An ingredient that causes oil to mix with water.

3. ____ A gelling agent made from animal bones and skin; it is a protein substance that, when mixed with liquid, forms a firm, jelly-like consistency.

4. ____ A salad that contains a gelling agent, liquid, and ingredients such as fruit, vegetables, protein foods, and grains; these salads are usually prepared in a mold.

5. ____ A mixture of oil and water.

Terms

A. agar agar
B. congealed salad
C. emulsifier
D. emulsion
E. gelatin

Name _____ Date _____ Period _____

CHAPTER 17 Great Grains

Activity A   Lesson 17.1

The Nitty-Gritty on Grains

Respond to the questions in the space provided.

1. Why are grains considered an important food for humans?
   _____
   _____

2. Label the parts of a grain.

A. _____

B. _____

C. _____

Wheat Foods Council

3. How is a whole-grain food different from a refined-grain food?
   _____
   _____

(Continued)

Name _____ Date _____ Period _____

4. How does the nutrient content of whole-grain foods compare with the nutrient content of refined-grain foods?
   _____
   _____

5. For each grain listed in the following table, identify its various forms or common foods made from the grain.

Grain	Forms and Common Foods
Wheat	
Corn	
Rice	
Oats	
Barley	
Rye	

6. Why are quinoa and wild rice called *psuedograins*?
   _____
   _____

Name _____ Date _____ Period _____

 **Activity B Lesson 17.1**

Grain Basics

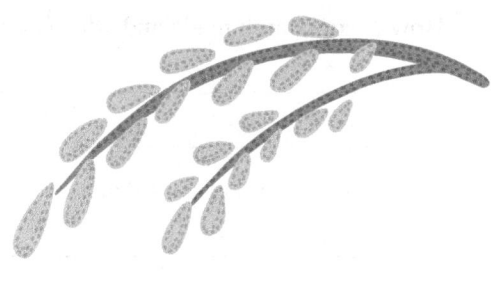

Use the reading from Lesson 17.1 to answer the questions that follow.

1. List five nutrients commonly found in grains.

   _____
   _____
   _____

2. Define the following terms:

   A. Bran

   _____
   _____

   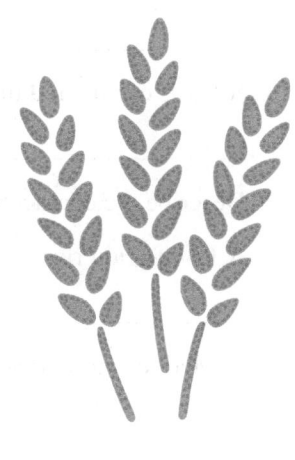

   B. Endosperm

   _____
   _____

   C. Germ

   _____
   _____

   D. Whole grain

   _____
   _____

   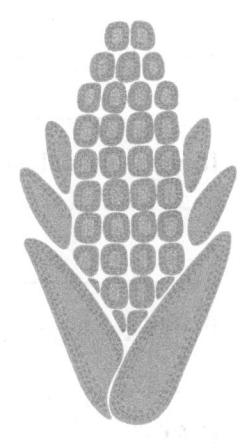

   E. Refined grain

   _____
   _____

   F. Enriched

   _____
   _____

3. Compare white flour with whole-wheat flour.

   _____
   _____
   _____
   _____

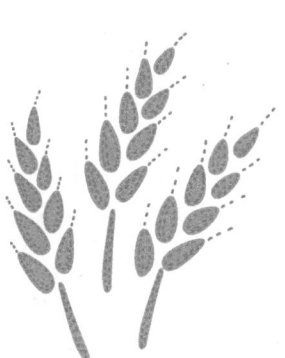

cosmaa/Shutterstock.com

(Continued)

Name _____ Date _____ Period _____

4. How is cornstarch made and what is it used for in cooking?
   _____
   _____

5. List the four types of corn that are considered grains and give an example of a food made from each.
   _____
   _____
   _____
   _____

6. What is considered the main food source for over half the people on Earth?
   _____

7. Describe the characteristics for each of the following after they are cooked:

   A. Long-grain rice
   _____

   B. Medium-grain rice
   _____

   C. Short-grain rice
   _____

8. Which type of rice discussed in the text has the highest nutritional content?
   _____

9. Identify one culinary use for each of the following grains:

   A. Oats
   _____

   B. Barley
   _____

   C. Rye
   _____

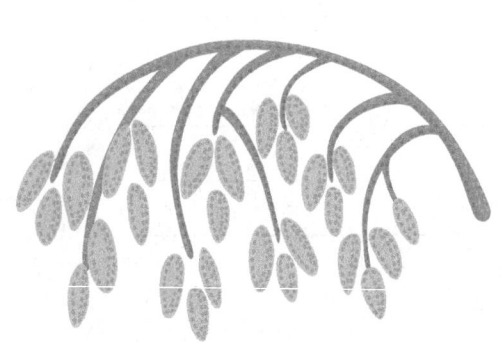
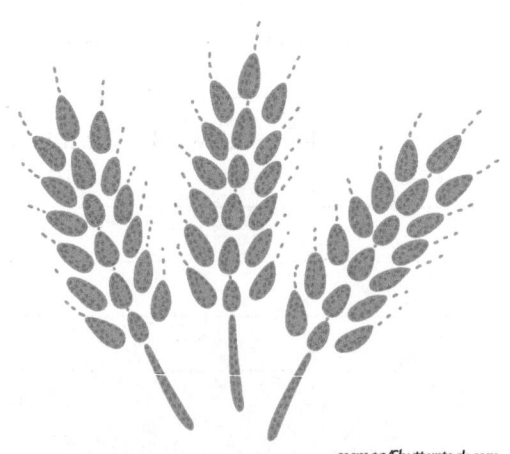

cosmaa/Shutterstock.com

84 Adventures in Food and Nutrition Workbook

Name _____ Date _____ Period _____

Activity C Lesson 17.2

Handling Grains

Use the reading from Lesson 17.2 to answer the questions that follow.

1. List one culinary use for breakfast cereals other than eating them as a meal or snack.
   _____

2. When buying breakfast cereal, should you purchase the box that is larger or the box that weighs more? Explain your answer.
   _____
   _____

3. List three forms in which rice can be purchased.
   _____
   _____

4. What are the two main ingredients in pasta?
   _____

5. List the five basic shapes of pasta.
   _____
   _____

6. What is usually added to pasta dough to create different colors and flavors?
   _____

7. What is added to flour to create self-rising flour?
   _____

8. Describe the best location to store most dried grain foods.
   _____
   _____

9. List three tips to preserve nutrients in grain foods during cooking.
   _____
   _____
   _____

10. Describe how flour and cornstarch act to thicken liquid.
    _____
    _____

Name _____ Date _____ Period _____

Activity D Chapter 17

New Terms Review

Read each definition and indicate which term is being described.

Definitions

1. ____ Food that has had the bran and germ removed to give it a smoother texture and help it stay fresh longer.
2. ____ The largest part of a grain kernel; contains mostly starch.
3. ____ Pasta that is cooked until it is tender but firm.
4. ____ Food that includes all three parts of the grain kernel.
5. ____ A process that occurs when starch granules absorb water, swell, and cause a liquid to get thicker.
6. ____ Food that has nutrients lost during processing added back to it.
7. ____ A grain kernel's tough outer coat.
8. ____ The smallest part of a grain kernel; contains most of the kernel's nutrients.

Terms

A. al dente
B. bran
C. endosperm
D. enriched
E. gelatinization
F. germ
G. refined grain
H. whole grain

Name _____ Date _____ Period _____

CHAPTER 18 Bountiful Breads

Activity A   Lesson 18.1

Let's Talk Bread!

Imagine you are being interviewed for a TV special about bread. Respond to the following interview questions as you would if asked during a TV interview.

1. How old is the bread-baking industry?
   _____
   _____

2. What nutrients are found in breads?
   _____
   _____

3. How are unleavened breads different from leavened breads?
   _____
   _____

4. What are examples of leavened breads and unleavened breads?
   _____
   _____

5. What makes leavened breads rise?
   _____
   _____

6. In what forms is bread sold?
   _____
   _____

7. What is your favorite type of bread? Why?
   _____
   _____

vectorlab2D/Shutterstock.com

Name _____ Date _____ Period _____

Activity B Lesson 18.2

Bread Basics

Answer the following questions in the space provided.

1. Indicate the function(s) of the bread ingredients in the table below:

Ingredient	Function(s)
Flour	
Liquid	
Sugar	
Fat	
Egg	
Leavening agent	

2. Compare batter with dough.

_____

_____

(Continued)

Name _____ Date _____ Period _____

3. Describe each of the mixing methods in the following table:

Method	Description
Muffin Method	
Biscuit Method	
Straight Dough Method	
Sponge Method	
Batter Method	
Rapid Mix Method	

4. Describe the Maillard reaction.

_____

_____

_____

Name _____ Date _____ Period _____

Activity C Chapter 18

New Terms Review

Read each definition and indicate which term is being described.

Definitions

1. ____ Ingredient or process that creates gas bubbles in baked goods, causing them to expand in size and become light and puffy.

2. ____ A mixture consisting of flour and liquid that is thick and stiff enough to be handled or kneaded.

3. ____ A sticky, elastic protein that forms when flour is mixed with liquid.

4. ____ A mixture consisting of flour and liquid that can be poured.

5. ____ Ingredient added to baked goods that produces carbon dioxide gas bubbles, which cause the baked goods to rise.

Terms

A. batter
B. dough
C. gluten
D. leavening
E. leavening agent

Name _____ Date _____ Period _____

CHAPTER 19 Luscious Legumes, Nuts, and Seeds

Activity A Lesson 19.1

Listen Up About Legumes

linear_design/Shutterstock.com

Answer the questions in the space provided.

1. Compare and contrast a legume with a pulse.

2. What nutrients are commonly found in legumes and pulses?

3. How do peanuts and soybeans differ from other legumes?

4. List the three main forms in which pulses can be purchased.

5. Which of the forms listed in #4 is the least expensive? Which takes the longest to prepare?

(Continued)

Name _____ Date _____ Period _____

6. What characteristics should you look for when selecting dried peas, beans, and lentils?

   _____
   _____
   _____
   _____

7. Explain how to prepare dried beans.

   _____
   _____
   _____
   _____

8. List three dishes that can be created with legumes.

   _____
   _____
   _____

9. Describe how to select wholesome, quality canned legumes.

   _____
   _____
   _____
   _____

10. How long can prepared legumes be stored in the refrigerator? the freezer?

    _____
    _____
    _____
    _____

Name _____ Date _____ Period _____

Activity B Lesson 19.2

Seeds of Knowledge

Answer the questions in the space provided.

1. What nutrients are found in nuts and seeds?

   _____
   _____
   _____
   _____

2. Why are nuts and seeds often used to make oils?

   _____
   _____
   _____
   _____

3. What characteristics should you look for when selecting nuts sold in bulk from large bins?

   _____
   _____
   _____
   _____

4. What factors affect the price of nuts and seeds?

   _____
   _____
   _____
   _____

5. How should nuts and seeds be stored?

   _____
   _____
   _____
   _____
   _____

Victoria Sergeeva/Shutterstock.com

(Continued)

Name _____ Date _____ Period _____

6. List three types of nut or seed flour.

   _____
   _____
   _____

7. What advice would you give a friend who is considering eliminating cow's milk from his or her diet and replacing it with nut and/or seed milks?

   _____
   _____
   _____
   _____
   _____
   _____

8. Explain how to toast nuts or seeds.

   _____
   _____
   _____
   _____
   _____

Victoria Sergeeva/Shutterstock.com

Name _____ Date _____ Period _____

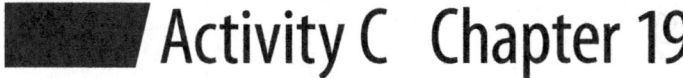 Activity C Chapter 19

Advice for a Vegetarian Diet

Your neighbor, Mr. Daughtry, is an animal lover. He wants to adopt a vegetarian diet because of his concern for the humane treatment of animals. He remembers that you are a Family and Consumer Sciences student and emails asking for your advice. Use your knowledge from Chapter 19 to give advice on using legumes, nuts, and seeds as part of a vegetarian diet. Be sure to discuss any special nutrient concerns and resources for menu planning.

From: Family & Consumer Sciences Student Expert <FCS@student.me>
To: Mr. Daughtry <daughtry@helpme.vit>

Subject: RE: Vegetarian Diet

Dear Mr. Daughtry,

_____
_____
_____
_____
_____
_____
_____
_____
_____
_____
_____
_____
_____
_____
_____
_____
_____
_____
_____
_____
_____
_____
_____
_____

Best,
Student Expert

Name _____ Date _____ Period _____

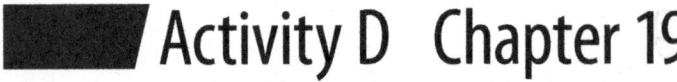 Activity D Chapter 19

New Terms Review

Read each definition and indicate which term is being described.

Definitions

1. ____ A soft, custard-like food made from soybeans.
2. ____ A person who does not eat meat, fish, or poultry.
3. ____ Any plant that produces edible seeds in a pod; also used to refer to the edible seeds produced by the plant.
4. ____ To start growing after a period of being dormant or not growing.
5. ____ The mature, dried seed harvested from the pod of a legume.

Terms

A. germinate
B. legume
C. pulse
D. tofu
E. vegetarian

Name _____ Date _____ Period _____

CHAPTER 20 Dairy Delights

Activity A Lesson 20.1

Dairy Details

Part 1
Complete each statement with a term from the list provided.

Statements

1. ____ Dairy products are rich in protein, _____, vitamin A, and riboflavin.
2. ____ A process that adds nutrients to a food that do not naturally occur in that food is called _____.
3. ____ Milk is fortified with _____.
4. ____ Milk and cream are mostly a watery liquid and _____.
5. ____ Health professionals believe drinking raw milk can result in _____.
6. ____ When fat is removed from milk, _____ is also removed.
7. ____ Milk contains a disaccharide called _____ that some people have trouble digesting.
8. ____ Flavored milks, such as chocolate milk, are higher in _____ than unflavored milk.
9. ____ Milk to which certain helpful bacteria have been added is called _____ milk.
10. ____ Clarifying butter removes the _____ and makes butter almost 100 percent fat.
11. ____ Pudding is thickened when the _____ granules gelatinize during cooking.
12. ____ Fresh cheeses have more _____ than aged cheeses.
13. ____ The first step in making cheese is to add a(n) _____ or acid to cause the solids to coagulate and form clumps.
14. ____ Sweet butter has no _____ added.

Terms

A. butterfat
B. calcium
C. calories
D. cultured
E. enzyme
F. foodborne illness
G. fortification
H. lactose
I. milk solids
J. moisture
K. salt
L. starch
M. vitamin A
N. vitamin D

(Continued)

Name _____ Date _____ Period _____

Part 2

Organize the following products by type in the table below.

Butter	Dry milk	Half-and-half	Pudding	UHT milk
Buttermilk	Eggnog	Ice cream	Queso blanco	Whole milk
Cheddar cheese	Evaporated milk	Kefir	Ricotta	Yogurt
Cottage cheese	Frozen yogurt	Lactose-free milk	Sour cream	

Dairy Product Type	Product(s)
Milk and Cream	
Cultured Milk Products	
Cheese	
Dairy Desserts	
Butter	

Organize the following cheeses by type in the table below.

Blue cheese	Cold pack cheese	Mozzarella cheese	Ricotta cheese
Brie cheese	Cottage cheese	Neufchatel cheese	Sap sago cheese
Cheddar cheese	Cream cheese	Parmesan cheese	Swiss cheese

Cheese Type	Cheese(s)
Fresh	
Aged	
Processed	

Name _____ Date _____ Period _____

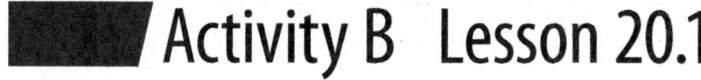 **Activity B Lesson 20.1**

Milk Matters

Provide a description for each dairy product in the following table and indicate how it can be used in meals.

Dairy Product	Description	Use
Buttermilk		
Dry Milk		
Evaporated Milk		
Frozen Milk Concentrate		
Half-and-Half		
Kefir		

(Continued)

Name _____ Date _____ Period _____

Dairy Product	Description	Use
Light Cream		
Sour Cream		
Sweetened Condensed Milk		
UHT Milk		
Whipping Cream		
Yogurt		

Name _____ Date _____ Period _____

Activity C Lesson 20.2

Avoiding a Dairy Disaster

1. List five factors to consider when selecting dairy products.
   _____
   _____
   _____

2. Complete the following table with storage guidelines for each type of dairy product listed.

Type	Storage
Milk and Cream	
Cultured Milk Products	
Dairy Desserts	
Cheese	
Butter	

3. For each of the dairy products in the following table, provide one tip for avoiding disasters when cooking.

Dairy Product	Tip
Milk	
Cheese	
Butter	

Indicate if the following statements about whipping cream are true or false.

4. ____ To get the greatest volume when whipping cream, choose cream with low fat content.

5. ____ If cream is overbeaten, it will separate into butter and whey.

6. ____ To sweeten whipped cream, add the sugar before you start whipping.

7. ____ Use brown sugar to sweeten whipped cream.

Name _____ Date _____ Period _____

Activity D Chapter 20

New Terms Review

Read each definition and indicate which term is being described.

Definitions

1. ____ Process that breaks the fat in milk or cream into tiny pieces and prevents the fat and watery liquid from separating.
2. ____ Dairy products produced by adding certain helpful bacteria to milk.
3. ____ The highest temperature a fat can reach before it smokes.
4. ____ Process that heats foods to a high temperature for a few seconds to kill harmful bacteria.
5. ____ The solid pieces in milk that can stick together to form lumps.
6. ____ Butter that has had its milk solids removed.
7. ____ Process used to remove milk solids from butter.
8. ____ A yellow-colored, bitter-tasting compound found naturally in some vegetables and fruits, coffee, and tea.
9. ____ To change from a liquid to a semi-solid or solid form.
10. ____ The liquid portion of milk that remains after curds form.

Terms

A. clarifying
B. coagulation
C. cultured milk product
D. curds
E. homogenization
F. pasteurization
G. ghee
H. smoke point
I. tannin
J. whey

Name _____ Date _____ Period _____

CHAPTER 21 Incredible Eggs

Activity A Lesson 21.1

Beneath the Shell

Follow the instructions in each part of this activity to check how well you understand eggs.

Part 1

Review the diagram and indicate the parts of the egg.

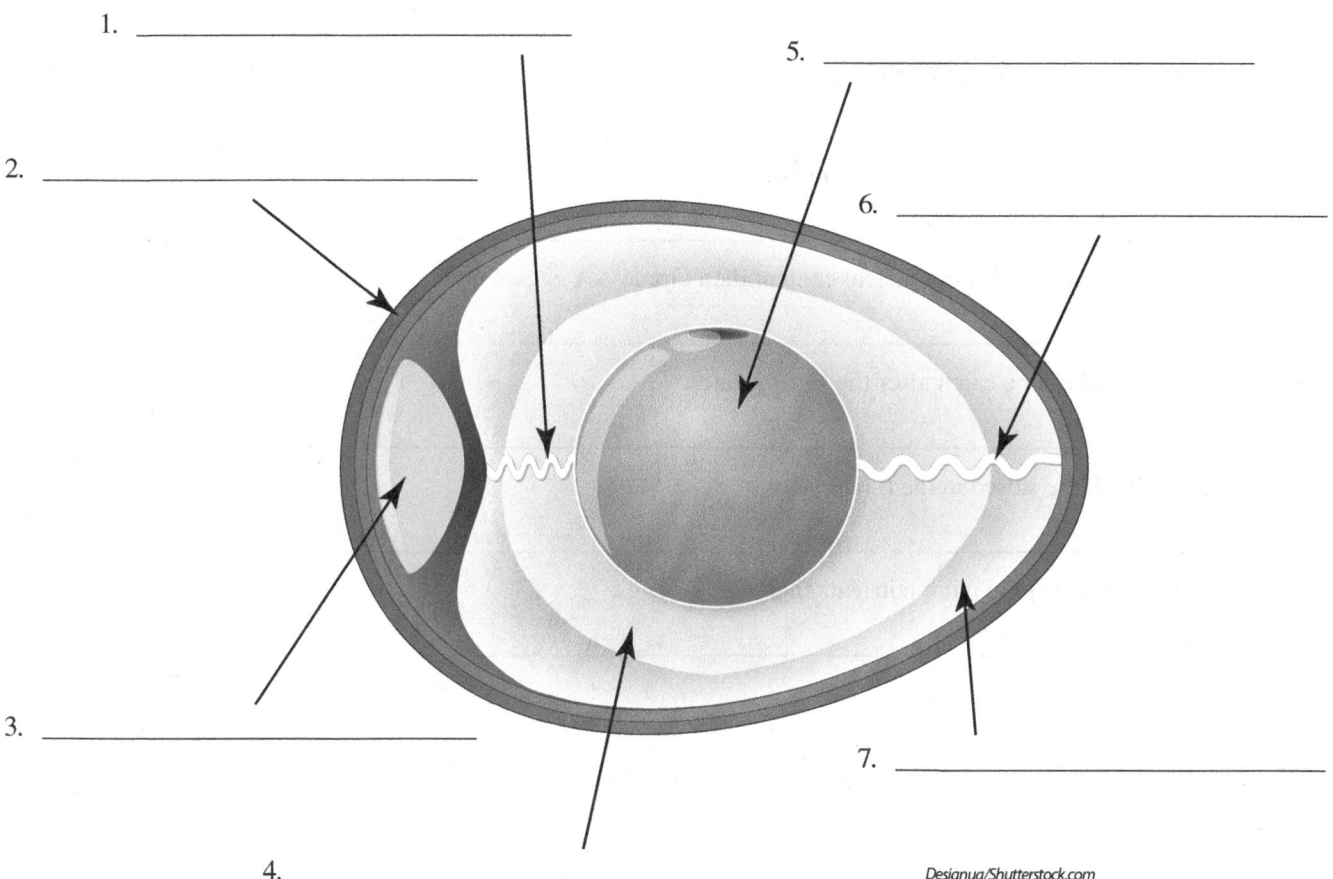

1. _____
2. _____
3. _____
4. _____
5. _____
6. _____
7. _____

Designua/Shutterstock.com

(Continued)

Name _____ Date _____ Period _____

Part 2

Indicate whether each of the following statements is true or false. If a statement is false, revise the statement to make it true in the space provided.

1. ____ One chicken egg has about 80 calories.
   _____

2. ____ Chicken eggs are a great source of fiber.
   _____

3. ____ All the fat and cholesterol of the egg is found in the yolk.
   _____

4. ____ The process by which eggs are graded is called *scoring*.
   _____

5. ____ The best-quality eggs are Grade A.
   _____

6. ____ Eggs are sized based on the weight of a dozen eggs.
   _____

7. ____ Most recipes are based on small eggs.
   _____

8. ____ The largest-sized eggs are called *jumbo*.
   _____

9. ____ Grade B eggs have lower nutrient content than Grade AA eggs.
   _____

10. ____ Eggs should *not* be eaten after the sell-by date.
    _____

11. ____ Eggs should be stored in the refrigerator.
    _____

12. ____ Organic eggs supply more nutrients than regular eggs.
    _____

Name _____ Date _____ Period _____

Activity B Lesson 21.2

Egg-Handling Intel

Use information from Lesson 21.2 to answer the following questions.

1. Why are eggs best stored in a covered container in the refrigerator?

   _____

   _____

   _____

2. Describe how to freeze eggs for long-term storage.

   _____

   _____

   _____

   _____

3. How can a person avoid the risk of foodborne illness from *Salmonella* from eggs?

   _____

   _____

4. What effect(s) does high cooking temperature and long cooking time have on eggs?

   _____

   _____

5. What grade egg should be used for a poached egg? Explain your answer.

   _____

   _____

   _____

6. What grade egg is best used for making a cake or cookies? Explain your answer.

   _____

   _____

   _____

7. List the four functions eggs perform in recipes.

   _____

   _____

   _____

Name _____ Date _____ Period _____

Activity C Chapter 21

New Terms Review

Read each definition and indicate which term is being described.

Definitions

1. ____ Shining a very bright light on eggs in order to judge their quality.
2. ____ A type of bacteria that can cause foodborne illness.
3. ____ Part of the egg that is clear and becomes white when cooked, also called *egg white*.
4. ____ White sting-like structure that holds the yolk in the middle of an egg.

Terms

A. albumen
B. candling
C. chalaza
D. *Salmonella*

Name _____ Date _____ Period _____

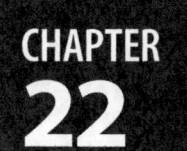

CHAPTER 22: Savory Seafood

Activity A Lesson 22.1

Fishy Business Profiles

Your "friends"—Frankie Finfish, Carlos Crustacean, Malia Mollusk, and Fatima Fatty Fish—want to create online business profiles that inform potential buyers (cooks) about who they are. Using what you learned in Lesson 22.1, create a description for each fish that includes information about how it differs from other seafood and why it is the preferred choice. Be creative!

Frankie Finfish

_____
_____
_____
_____
_____
_____
_____
_____

Carlos Crustacean

_____
_____
_____
_____
_____
_____
_____
_____
_____

davooda/Shutterstock.com

(Continued)

Name _____ Date _____ Period _____

Malia Mollusk

_____
_____
_____
_____
_____
_____
_____
_____
_____

Fatima Fatty Fish

_____
_____
_____
_____
_____
_____
_____
_____
_____

davooda/Shutterstock.com

Name _____ Date _____ Period _____

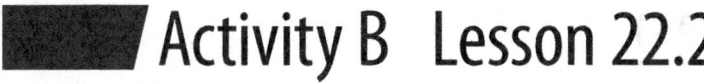 Activity B Lesson 22.2

Name That Cut

Match the fish cut with its corresponding image.

Images

1. ____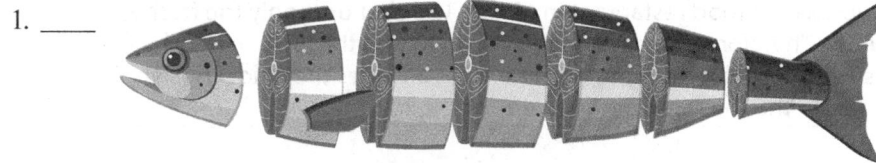

2. ____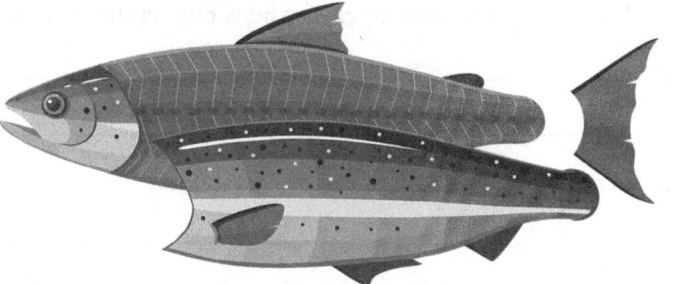

3. ____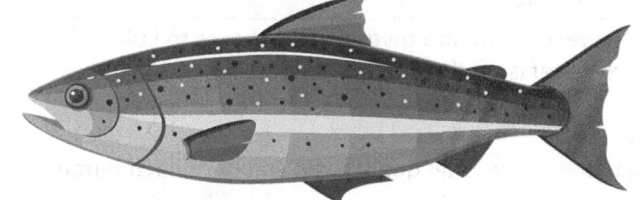

4. ____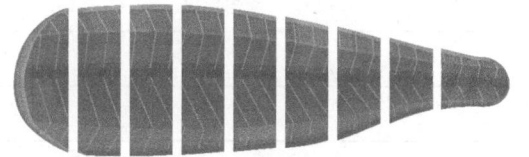

5. ____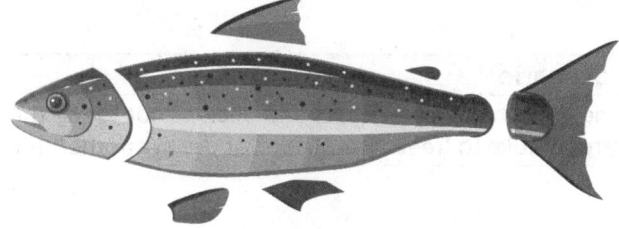

6. ____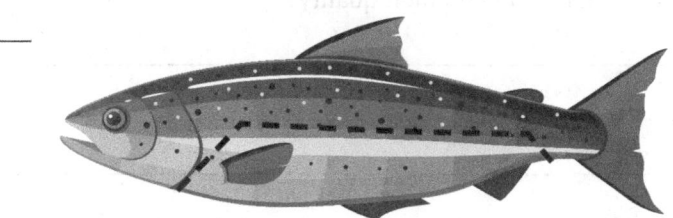

Fish Cuts

A. drawn fish
B. dressed fish
C. fish fillet
D. fish steaks
E. fish sticks
F. whole fish

De-Frozen/Shutterstock.com

Name _____ Date _____ Period _____

Activity C Lesson 22.2

Seafood Sourcing

Read the scenarios and answer the questions that follow.

Scenario
Rashaud is the food buyer for an upscale seafood restaurant in Maine. The chef uses only the freshest ingredients in her seafood restaurant. Therefore, she has hired Rashaud to visit the local seafood market every morning to buy fresh seafood. This morning, the chef's list includes the following: whole rainbow trout, salmon steaks, oysters in the shell, and live lobster.

1. What factors should Rashaud look for when selecting his purchases to ensure he is buying the freshest seafood?

_____
_____
_____
_____

Scenario
After buying the seafood, Rashaud returns to the restaurant and gives the purchases to Luke, who is responsible for storing the fresh seafood until the chef is ready to begin preparation.

2. Explain how Luke should store each of the purchases to ensure the quality and safety of each purchase is maintained.

_____
_____
_____
_____

Scenario
When the chef arrives at the restaurant, she reviews Rashaud's purchases and decides not to use the salmon steaks on the day's menu. The chef instructs Luke to freeze the steaks for use at another time.

3. How should Luke prepare the salmon steaks for freezing to maintain their quality?

_____
_____
_____
_____

(Continued)

Name _____ Date _____ Period _____

Scenario
The next day, the chef sends Rashaud back to the market to purchase fish for the dinner special. The dinner special is always a limited quantity and sells out quickly. The chef wants Rashaud to purchase just enough to serve 20 people. Rashaud will decide which fish to purchase once he sees what is available at the market and will calculate how much to buy based on the cut.

4. Calculate how many ounces Rashaud should buy for each option that follows. Show your work.

   A. Seafood without skin, bones, or shells:

   _____

   _____

   B. Fresh finfish fillets:

   _____

   _____

   C. Dressed fish:

   _____

   _____

   D. Whole fish:

   _____

   _____

   E. Clams:

   _____

   _____

Name _____ Date _____ Period _____

Activity D Chapter 22

New (and Other) Terms Review

Read each definition and indicate which term is being described.

Definitions

1. ____ Animals that have a backbone or spinal column that helps support their bodies.
2. ____ Seafood that has a backbone and fins.
3. ____ Animals that do not have a backbone or spinal column.
4. ____ To preserve a food by removing its moisture using processes like smoking, salting, drying, and pickling.
5. ____ Seafood with no bones; most have a hard shell.
6. ____ Shellfish that have been removed from their shell.

Terms

A. curing
B. finfish
C. invertebrate
D. shellfish
E. shucked
F. vertebrate

Name _____ Date _____ Period _____

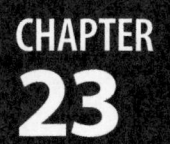

CHAPTER 23: Marvelous Meat and Poultry

Activity A Lesson 23.1

Meat and Poultry Basics

Part 1

Indicate whether each of the following statements is true or false. If a statement is false, revise the statement to make it true in the space provided.

1. ____ The four major parts that make up the structure of meat are muscle, fat, water, and bone.

2. ____ Connective tissue can make meat tender.

3. ____ The fat in poultry is found mostly just below the skin.

4. ____ A donut-shaped bone in a piece of meat indicates the meat is from the animal's rib.

5. ____ Meat is rich in iron and zinc.

6. ____ The fat found in meat is primarily unsaturated fat.

7. ____ A meat that has been stamped *US Inspected* means it is safe to eat.

8. ____ Meat cuts from well-exercised muscles are more tender than cuts from muscles that get little exercise.

9. ____ As a chicken gets older, its meat becomes more tender.

10. ____ Dressed poultry has had its feathers, blood, and part of its digestive system removed.

(Continued)

Name _____ Date _____ Period _____

Part 2

Match each letter on the diagram with its corresponding primal cut.

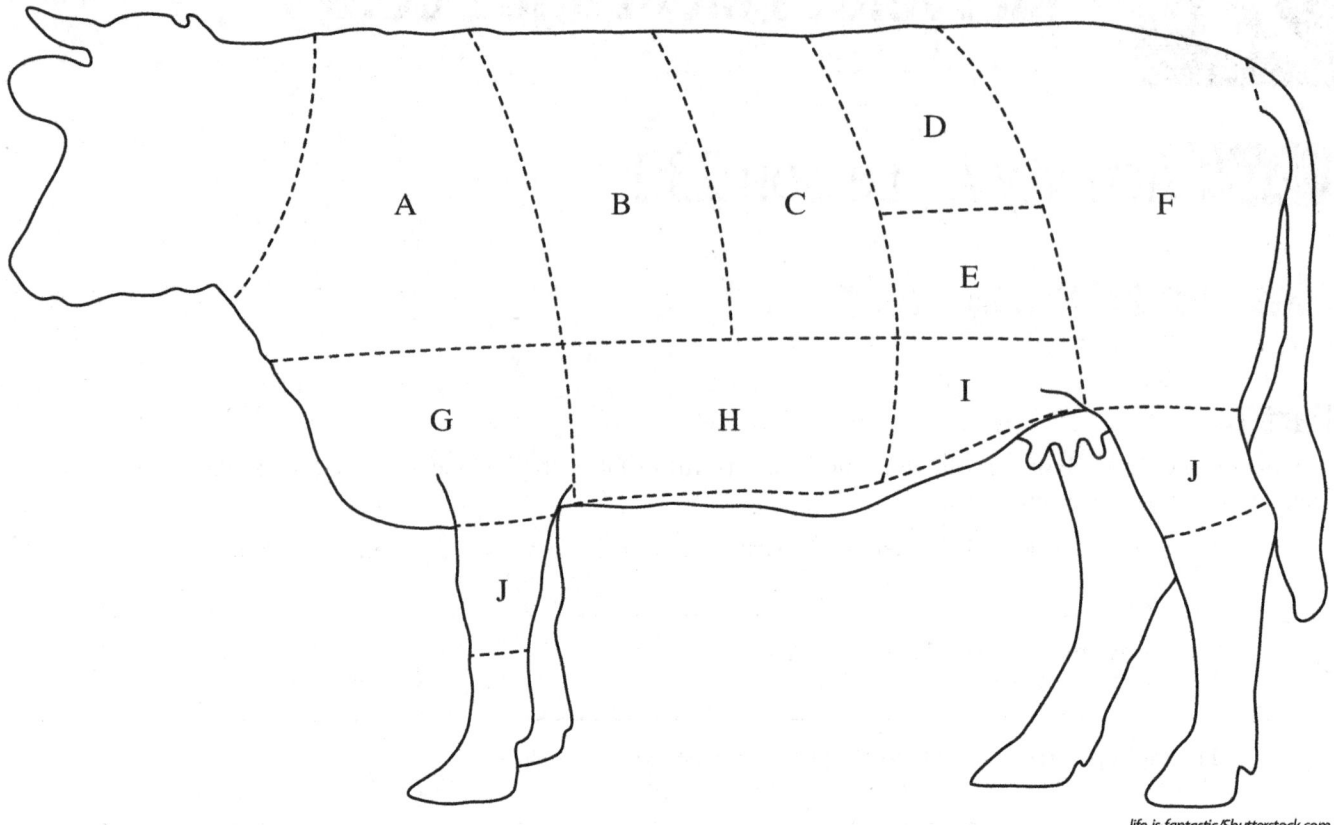

11. ____ Short plate
12. ____ Round
13. ____ Shank
14. ____ Chuck
15. ____ Rib
16. ____ Short loin
17. ____ Sirloin
18. ____ Flank
19. ____ Bottom sirloin
20. ____ Brisket

Name _____ Date _____ Period _____

Activity B Lesson 23.2

Handling Meats and Poultry

Use information from Lesson 23.2 to answer the following questions.

1. List four factors that affect the price of fresh meats and poultry.
   _____
   _____

2. Describe what to look for when selecting frozen meats.
   _____
   _____

3. How should raw meat and poultry be stored in the refrigerator? Explain your answer.
   _____
   _____

4. Why should meat be taken out of the refrigerator and allowed to warm slightly before cooking?
   _____
   _____

5. Why do higher-quality grades and tender cuts require less cooking time?
   _____
   _____

6. If you are cooking a large roast and want a final temperature of 145°F, at what temperature should you remove it from the oven to account for carryover cooking? Show your work.
   _____
   _____

7. If you are asked to cook a large cut of meat that is tough, what type of cooking method would you choose? Explain your answer.
   _____
   _____

Name _____ Date _____ Period _____

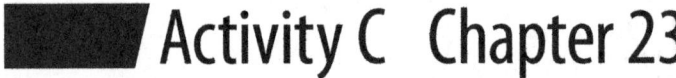 Activity C Chapter 23

New (and Other) Terms Review

Read each definition and indicate which term is being described.

Definitions

1. ____ The organs of an animal such as liver, kidney, heart, tongue, and brains.
2. ____ Streaks of fat that run through meat; makes meat tender and juicy.
3. ____ The part of the bone where blood cells are made.
4. ____ Ingredient used in cured meats that gives them a pink color, adds flavor, helps preserve them, and prevents the foodborne illness called *botulism*.
5. ____ Long, thin tissue that holds muscles together.
6. ____ The direction that the fascicles and fibrils run in meat.

Terms

A. connective tissue
B. grain
C. marbling
D. marrow
E. sodium nitrite
F. variety meats

Name _____ Date _____ Period _____

CHAPTER 24 Delicious Desserts

Activity A Lesson 24.1

Conquering Cake

Complete the table that follows by describing each ingredient's function in cake baking.

Ingredient	Function
Baking soda, baking powder, steam, or air	
Flour	
Egg	
Sugar	
Fat	
Liquid	
Flavoring	

(Continued)

Name _____ Date _____ Period _____

Read the following statements and use an "S" to indicate if the statement describes shortened cake and an "F" if the statement describes foam cake.

1. _____ Little or no fat content.
2. _____ Fat content from butter or shortening.
3. _____ Leavened with whipped egg whites.
4. _____ Leavened with baking powder or baking soda.
5. _____ Thin, evenly colored crust.
6. _____ Thin, tender, golden brown crust that looks rough and slightly cracked.
7. _____ Crust feels a little sticky.
8. _____ Smooth and rounded top crust.

Indicate if each of the following statements is true or false.

9. _____ The first step of the quick-mix method is to cream the fat and sugar until they are light and fluffy.
10. _____ The conventional method for mixing cakes requires three bowls.
11. _____ A shortened cake with pale color, tough crust, and coarse crumb with tunnels running through the interior has been undermixed.
12. _____ Cream of tartar strengthens foams made from egg whites.
13. _____ Dark metal cake pans increase baking time and produce a cake with a pale crust.
14. _____ Cake pans made from thinner-gauge metal produce a higher-quality cake than pans made from thicker-gauge metal.
15. _____ When baking cakes in dark metal or glass pans, the heat indicated in the recipe should be lowered by 25°F (14°C) and round pans should be used.
16. _____ When baking foam cakes, the cake pans should be greased.
17. _____ The oven should be preheated to help trap the leavening gases in the cake.
18. _____ A cake with crust that is too brown, cracked, and formed a peak in the middle is an indication the oven was too cool.
19. _____ A sign that cakes are done baking is when they start to pull away from the sides of the pan.
20. _____ A shortened cake should be allowed to cool completely before removing it from the pan.
21. _____ Cake should be slightly warm when it is frosted.
22. _____ Cakes cannot be frozen.

Name _____ Date _____ Period _____

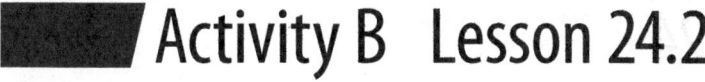 **Activity B Lesson 24.2**

Deciphering Desserts

Read each phrase and indicate which type of cookie is being described.

Statements

1. ____ Dough is rolled out and cut into shapes; examples include sandwich cookies, shortbread cookies, and sugar cookies.
2. ____ Soft cookie dough is spread in a pan, baked, cooled, and cut into cookies; examples include brownies, blondies, and date bars.
3. ____ Stiff dough is pushed through a press to form cookies; examples include spritz cookies and lemon crisps.
4. ____ Spoonfuls of dough are placed onto a cookie sheet and baked; examples include oatmeal cookies and chocolate chip cookies.
5. ____ Dough is shaped into a roll, wrapped, chilled, cut into slices, and baked; an example is pinwheel cookies.
6. ____ Dough is shaped by hand into shapes such as balls or crescents; an example is peanut butter cookies.

Cookie Types

A. bar
B. drop
C. molded
D. pressed
E. refrigerator
F. rolled

Use information from Lesson 24.2 to answer the following questions.

7. List three tips for making cookies.

   _____
   _____
   _____

8. How do plain pastry piecrusts and puff pastry piecrusts differ?

   _____
   _____

9. Describe the three ingredients needed to make the most flaky piecrust.

   _____
   _____

10. When making a piecrust, why is the size the fat is cut into important?

    _____
    _____

Name _____ Date _____ Period _____

Activity C Chapter 24

New Terms Review

Read each definition and indicate which term is being described.

Definitions

1. _____ Starch from cassava used to thicken desserts.
2. _____ Dough that is lightly rolled flat and remains flat during baking.
3. _____ Mixing method used for shortened cakes in which fat and sugar are creamed together, the eggs are added, and sifted dry ingredients are added alternately with the liquid ingredients.
4. _____ Cake that contains fat such as butter or shortening.
5. _____ Cake that contains no fat; sometimes called *unshortened cake*.
6. _____ Dough that is folded and rolled many times before baking, which causes it to increase in size up to eight times.
7. _____ Interior of a baked product.
8. _____ Mixing method used for shortened cakes in which dry ingredients are sifted into a mixing bowl, the fat and liquid are added, and then the eggs are added.
9. _____ Cake made by blending fat with beaten egg whites, cake flour, and leavening agents.

Terms

A. chiffon cake
B. conventional method
C. crumb
D. foam cake
E. plain pastry
F. puff pastry
G. quick-mix method
H. shortened cake
I. tapioca

Name _____ Date _____ Period _____

A Career to Consider

Activity A   Lesson 25.1

Career Reflection

There are many career opportunities in food and nutrition. For this assignment, reflect on the information from Lesson 25.1 as well as your own personal qualities to answer the questions in the spaces provided.

1. Identify one career discussed in this lesson that you could imagine pursuing. Explain why this career appeals to you.

    _____
    _____

2. What skills or personal qualities do you possess that would make this a suitable career choice?

    _____
    _____

3. What fears or hesitations do you have about pursuing this career?

    _____
    _____

4. What actions could you take to overcome those fears or hesitations?

    _____
    _____

5. Does the idea of being an entrepreneur interest you? Explain your answer.

    _____
    _____

6. Identify one food- or nutrition-related interest that you have and how you could turn it into a business. Be creative!

    _____
    _____

Copyright Goodheart-Willcox Co., Inc.
May not be reproduced or posted to a publicly accessible website.

Name _____ Date _____ Period _____

Activity B Lesson 25.2

Your Vision for a Career

Answer the following questions in the space provided.

1. What type of a daily routine do you hope to have in a career?

   _____
   _____
   _____
   _____

2. What level of responsibility do you want: Working under direct supervision? Supervising the work of others?

   _____
   _____
   _____
   _____

3. What type of working conditions do you want?

   _____
   _____
   _____
   _____

4. Do you imagine traveling for work? If so, how much?

   _____
   _____
   _____
   _____

5. Do you plan to pursue education beyond high school? If so, what kind?

   _____
   _____
   _____
   _____

(Continued)

Name _____ Date _____ Period _____

6. What would give you satisfaction in a career—helping others, financial gain, work-life balance, other?
_____
_____
_____
_____
_____

7. What skills do you have that would be important to include on a résumé?
_____
_____
_____
_____
_____

8. What qualities do you have that employers expect from employees?
_____
_____
_____
_____
_____

9. Based on your answers to questions 1–8, what career discussed in Lesson 25.1 interests you? Is this the same career you identified in question 1 in Activity A? If not, explain why your answer changed.
_____
_____
_____
_____
_____

10. Use an online career source (see Figure 25.9) to learn more about the career identified in question 9. Then list three goals to help you plan and prepare for this career.
_____
_____
_____
_____
_____

Name _____ Date _____ Period _____

Activity C Chapter 25

New Terms Review

Read each definition and indicate which term is being described.

Definitions

1. ____ Aims you want to achieve.
2. ____ A document that summarizes your personal information, education, work experience, and references; provides the information employers need to decide if your qualifications match their needs.
3. ____ The use of words to send or receive information; includes both written and spoken words.
4. ____ A series of related jobs you hold over a period of time in a chosen field.
5. ____ Beliefs and ideas that are important to you.
6. ____ A person who organizes, manages, and assumes responsibility for a business.
7. ____ People an employer can call to ask about your abilities as a worker.
8. ____ The process of selecting a logical choice from the available options.
9. ____ The sending of a message without the use of words.
10. ____ Focusing on the message that is being communicated both verbally and nonverbally with the goal of understanding the speaker's message.
11. ____ A series of jobs in the same field through which you can advance.
12. ____ The sending or receiving of information.

Terms

A. active listening
B. career
C. career ladder
D. communication
E. decision-making
F. entrepreneur
G. goals
H. nonverbal communication
I. references
J. résumé
K. values
L. verbal communication